HANDBOOK

—— OF ——

NATURAL THERAPIES

Exploring the Spiral of Healing

by Marcia Starck

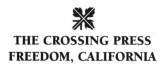

THE CROSSING PRESS
FREEDOM, CALIFORNIA

For information on bulk purchases or group discounts for this and other
Crossing Press titles, please contact our Special Sales Manager at 800-777-1048.
Visit our Website on the Internet at: www.crossingpress.com

Healing and medicine are two very different disciplines, and the law requires the following disclaimer. The information in this book is not medicine but healing, and it does not constitute medical advice. In case of serious illness consult the practitioner of your choice.

Library of Congress Cataloging-in-Publication Data
Starck, Marcia.
    Handbook of natural therapies : exploring the spiral of healing / by Marcia Starck.
       p. cm.
    Includes index.
    ISBN 0-89594-869-9 (pbk.)
    1. Naturopathy—Handbooks, manuals, etc. 2. Self-care, Health—Handbooks, manuals,etc. 3. Therapeutics—Handbooks, manuals, etc. 4. Therapeutics—Popular works.
I. Title.
RZ440.S74 1998
615.5'35—dc21
                                                                 98-4962
                                                                CIP

You may contact Marcia Starck, Medical Astrologer, at:
Earth Medicine Ways
P.O. Box 5435
Santa Fe, NM 87502
505-473-1464

This book is dedicated to the memory of my father,
Paul Rittenberg,
whose death at an early age inspired me
to explore the path of Natural Healing.

ACKNOWLEDGMENTS

I wish to acknowledge several people whose editorial assistance was instrumental in bringing this book into being. First, Judith Pynn for her inspiration in helping to map out the format of the book. Secondly, Miriam Avins whose editing made the book more cohesive and understandable. Third, Jill Schettler and Cyndi Barnes of *The Crossing Press* for overseeing all the details, and fourth, Elaine Goldman Gill, my publisher, for her flexibility in allowing this project to be birthed.

Thanks to the Art Department at *The Crossing Press* for designing this book and its cover.

To the many friends whose energy supported me during the writing of this book, I am truly grateful.

TABLE OF CONTENTS

PREFACE

Before compiling this book, I asked myself the question, "Why another book on natural healing techniques?" My answer is that alternative healing has changed its focus and scope in recent years, and continues to evolve as more people explore, use, and benefit from these modalities.

The first bloom of the natural healing movement (in the 1960s) emphasized organic foods and products, bodywork therapies such as massage, and acupuncture and Oriental healing systems. More recently, vibrational therapies such as homeopathy, flower essences and aromas, and magnetic healing techniques are entering the mainstream of alternative healing as are therapies that focus on the mind-body connection. Many people are also using Shamanic techniques such as dreamwork, guided imagery, and Reichian breathwork.

The sheer abundance and variety of natural therapies available today can cause confusion. One purpose of this book is to clarify the role of many alternative therapies, both for people who have been using such therapies for years, and for people who have not yet been introduced to alternative medicine.

The organization of this book is also different from other books on natural healing. I have started with the modalities that work with the electrical vibrations of the universe, to those that focus on how our minds and emotions affect our health, to those that emphasize the physical interactions among our cells. These modalities form a continuum or spiral of healing. All parts of this continuum are necessary for true health, and I hope that this way of presenting the information will help you on your own journey of healing.

—Marcia Starck
Santa Fe, New Mexico
October, 1997

INTRODUCTION

For many, modern medical science is of little use; its insistence on chemical drugs to treat physical symptoms has created more toxicity in the body and more new "diseases" than have ever been known. Many people are looking to alternative (or complementary) medicine for answers to their health problems. Alternative medicine focuses on the body's ability to heal itself and the need for people to live in harmony with the natural world; it also uses remedies that are derived from unprocessed natural substances.

Unfortunately, the field of alternative medicine has grown so large that it has spawned confusion and often skepticism. The proponents of each type of healing art or therapy claim that their particular focus is the key to healing. For example, acupuncture focuses on the flow of "chi" or life force through meridians in our bodies. Chiropractic practitioners claim that misalignment of the vertebrae reduces the ability of the nerves to function properly, and can lead to a wide variety of symptoms. Macrobiotic teachers believe that the solution to health problems is to eat the correct balance of yin and yang foods. Those who heal with gems and crystals focus on how the light energy specific to each stone can affect our own energy.

How is one to choose among such disparate therapies? And are these therapies related to each other within some larger scheme? I have discussed these two issues in this book. I believe natural healing techniques address different causes of disease and different possibilities for healing. And I do believe that these techniques are related within a larger scheme and have so organized this book.

I begin with the work of an extraordinary man, Paracelsus von Hohenheim, a Swiss medical doctor and alchemist who lived in the fifteenth century. This scientist and mystic is called the father of modern medicine. He devoted his life to research in the healing arts by exploring the fields of animal magnetism, alchemy, folk medicine, astrology, and Kabbalism. He visited Constantinople to learn the practices of the Dervishes and Sufis. He was a practical person, concerned with the recovery of the sick, rather than the perpetuation of orthodox procedures in use at the time. Paracelsus is credited with the discovery of hydrogen and nitrogen. He developed methods for the administration of mercury in the treatment of certain diseases, established a correlation between cretinism and goiter, and introduced the use of mineral baths. He studied the writings of Pythagoras and Plato. He integrated the healing methods used before his time: vibrational healing, Traditional Chinese Medicine, biofeedback, herbology, dietary regimes, and colonic irrigation.

FUNDAMENTAL IDEAS OF PARACELSUS

Like many natural healers throughout the ages, Paracelsus emphasized our oneness with the universe. Healers who focus on specific bodily mechanisms focus on the need to give our bodies appropriate foods and other natural substances. Practitioners in the more esoteric branches of healing focus on the energy in each thing on earth and in the sky. Paracelsus' term for such energy is "universal life force." This is a concept that has been used by all cultures—it is the "chi" of Traditional Chinese Medicine, the "prana" of Ayurveda, the "mana" of the Polynesians, and the "orenda" of certain tribal cultures.

Paracelsus wrote that we are connected to the total universe by energy correspondences. Everything that lives—from the tiniest organism in a drop of water, to a small herb, to a huge animal—is a focal point of universal life energy. Paracelsus advised physicians to examine "the celestial constellations of the sky, the terrestrial constellations upon the earth, and the physiological constellations within man." "For every star in the sky there is a flower in the meadow, and for each ray that comes out of space, there is an integration on every level of structure." He pointed out that there are integrations of cosmic forces in the mineral, vegetable, animal, and human kingdoms. The knowledge of astrology and astronomical phenomena is very important in the healing realm; we need to understand the cosmic influences that are affecting all living matter before we can look specifically at each human being.

A more modern formulation of this idea was developed in reaction to the *Gaia hypothesis* of the 1970s. The Gaia hypothesis claims that the earth is a living, breathing organism who feels the decimation, pillage, and rape of her being; she fights back through volcanoes, earthquakes, and flooding. Similarly, humans experience the actions and thoughts of others, and take on bodily symptoms such as raging fevers, broken bones, and swollen extremities. In this view, prayer and meditation, along with an understanding of why we have developed the particular symptoms, can initiate the process of healing and help us to restore our vital force.

For Paracelsus, all growing things, through their structure, form, color, and aroma, reveal their particular use to humans. This idea has been the starting point for herbalists, homeopaths, those who work with flower and gem essences, and aromatherapists. Homeopathy has incorporated the idea physically in remedies like *nux vomica*, the nut that makes you vomit. Nux vomica is full of strychnine and is poisonous if eaten. The homeopathic remedy, how-ever, is used for getting rid of toxins and poisons in the body. The same con-cept is used psychologically in the remedy *pulsatilla,* which means pulsating or changing direction with the wind. Those individuals whose constitution is pulsatilla are often changeable and soft like the flower.

Paracelsus described the universal life force as light, distinguishing it from what he called darkness, the inner light or light of the soul. Darkness supports the powers that are uniquely human, particularly intuition. That is why many traditional systems of healing include meditation, along with physical cleans-ing, diet, and herbal remedies in order to enhance the body's intuitive wis-doms. Today, prayer, meditation, and visualization have come to be accepted as viable techniques.

Not surprisingly, Paracelsus felt that a physician must be more than a sci-entist; the physician to him was a holy man, "a servant of the light which flows from the heart of the Infinite." Similarly, healers in many cultures—the med-icine man, shaman, or healer-priest—not only know the native plants and can set a bone, but also carry the spiritual energy necessary for healing. The revival of ancient healing systems and their spiritual philosophies at the end of the twentieth century is testimony to the need we Westerners have to re-connect with the type of physician Paracelsus describes. There is a vast re-surgence of interest in the wisdom of the Mayans, Incans, and Toltecs. Many are exploring Asian shamanism with their studies of Traditional Chinese Medicine, Tibetan medicine, and Ayurveda. Still others are reclaiming Celtic knowledge and the Druidic priesthood.

Paracelsus believed that each disease is an organism with its own energy. Diseases develop through an orderly sequence of symptoms, they will attack various parts of the body, and some survive like parasites in the body. He felt that diseases arise from one or more of five basic causes and insisted that the physician be aware of all of these causes so that he could judge the proportions of each cause in contributing to a particular illness or imbalance.

The First Cause

The first cause of disease is "sidereal and astral influences acting upon the invisible etheric or vital body of man." (The *etheric body,* which guides the cell's activities, can be thought of as the home of the universal life force. See Chapter 2 for a fuller discussion.) These influences set in motion various vibrations which are diffused throughout the physical body and are possible causes of imbalance. Paracelsus explains that there are mutations of sidereal forces and magnetic rays which operate on the magnetic field of the earth, affecting the health of humans. An example of this might be a comet some-where in the solar system, especially if it moves close to the earth's magnetic field, causing increased vibrations which would affect an individual's nervous system. This phenomenon happened in July 1995 when Jupiter was hit by a comet. Observing the changes on Jupiter's surface through telescopes and binoculars, we also witnessed strange weather patterns here on Earth. The increased electrical energies led to more physical imbalances and illnesses. Understanding how the comet was influencing us was crucial to not becoming a victim of psycho-physical imbalances.

By understanding cosmic influences, we can remain healthy by affecting our own magnetic fields. For example, Paracelsus writes of the magnetic field surrounding the endocrine glands, which store and regulate the distribution of energy. If we deplete our resources too rapidly when no restoring energies are available, we may find ourselves fatigued or devitalized.

Paracelsus believed that epidemics are not cured or terminated by medical skill, but may be caused and ended by mutations in the atmosphere, the configuration of planets, and broad psychic disturbances that might arise from war, panic, or fanaticism. According to Paracelsus, humans possess the capability to store up psychic and spiritual energy so that they may retain their life force during "psychic mutations of nature." This idea is similar to the concept in shamanic cultures of learning to preserve personal power.

It is also helpful to know our own cosmic blueprint known as the astrological horoscope. A horoscope is like a road map for our lives in that it shows our personal areas of sensitivity and strength. Through the study of Medical Astrology, we can become aware of which organs and body systems are prone to weakness and work to strengthen those areas through particular herbs, supplements, homeopathic remedies, exercise, and various therapies such as acupuncture or bodywork. We can also understand the timing of certain planetary influences that account for our feeling very tired or nervous or our experiencing pain in a certain area of the body. Knowing that there is a cosmic reason for all imbalance and disease can alleviate anxiety and worry as to what is causing the symptom as well as guilt, which often takes the form of blaming ourselves for eating the wrong foods, for not exercising, or for holding back certain emotions. Sometimes, even when we do everything that will, we think, help us maintain our life force, we still manifest symptoms due to the way the planets are transiting through our birth charts. Understanding planetary causes can provide us with ways to go about healing the imbalance; it can also give us an idea of when the particular symptom might disappear if we take responsibility and do the healing required.

The Second Cause

Paracelsus writes that disobedience to "religious, moral, and ethical laws" can lead to disease. Here he is alluding to disobeying one's conscience or of breaking natural law. He speaks of spiritual causes of sickness that might be present before birth. For example, if someone is born with a serious disease and must spend much time in healing and working within strong physical limitations, the disease is obviously related to what the individual has done before being born into this life, as well as spiritual work in future lives. For example, it may be that there is some lesson in learning how to live with a disability in order to fulfill a particular soul plan. Or someone who has enjoyed a position of power and control over others in a past life might come back in a weakened physical body in order to experience vulnerability. (This could also happen in the same life if one loses physical abilities through a stroke or accident.)

The Third Cause

Paracelsus' third cause of disease is psychological; imbalances of the mind and emotions lead not only to discomfort of the body but to ailments that are difficult to diagnose and treat. For example, he explained that violent emotion can cause miscarriage, anger can cause jaundice, and grief can depress a being so much that it dies. Conversely, joy can stimulate sluggish functions and help to restore health.

Such psychosomatic causes of illness and healing are being explored today. In his book, *The Stress of Life*, Dr. Hans Selye uses his experiments with rats to explain how the hormonal system and other biochemical processes adapt to stressful conditions in one's job or family life. He also showed that the kidneys are affected by stress, and why blood pressure may be high during stressful periods. Dr. Selye explained how mal-functioning of the liver may lead to abnormal blood sugar levels and difficulty in de-toxifying chemical substances in the environment.

Traditional systems of medicine also draw connections between emotional states and the diseases of specific organs. For example, in Traditional Chinese Medicine, the liver and gall bladder are associated with the element Wood, the season spring, and anger. Those with diseases of these organs, such as diabetes and cirrhosis of the liver, tend to hold back their anger, and often their tears as well. The small intestine and heart relate to joy and sorrow, the element Fire, and summer. Those who carry much sadness and sorrow within them often have problems with the cardiovascular system. The spleen and stomach are associated with sympathy, the Earth element, and late summer. Those with stomach ulcers and those lacking hydrochloric acid seem to have difficulty expressing sympathy and emotions in general. Lung and large intestine problems are correlated with worry and grief; they are related to the element Air and autumn. Those who tend to worry a lot, those who hold a lot of grief within, as well as those who are very mental, experience problems as bronchitis, asthma, and pneumonia in addition to digestive problems such as colitis, flatulence, and indigestion. The fluid mucus is related to these organs and when one gets in touch with long-standing grief, a lot of mucus may be released from the lungs. The kidney and bladder signify fear, the Water element, and winter. Cystitis, nephritis, and other kidney and bladder problems related to fear often create an imbalance in terms of heat and cold and alkaline and acid. Ayurveda and other systems also relate particular organs and body systems to specific emotions.

The Fourth Cause

Paracelsus' fourth cause of disease is the introduction into the body of various impurities, poisons, or hurtful substances—including drugs and medications for the alleviation of disease.

In Paracelsus' day, hygiene and hygienic food preparation were an important issue, and proper standards of sanitation and cleanliness are still an issue in most countries today. A more important issue today, however, involves toxic chemicals being added to foods as preservatives, or pesticides sprayed on fruits and vegetables. A whole new field of medicine focusing on environmental illness has sprung up.

Paracelsus was indeed a prophet when he speculated that drugs and medications would be used for the alleviation of disease. Four centuries later, the drug industry has become a huge obstacle to any type of natural healing, since, in alleviating one symptom or in attacking what conventional medicine understands as the cause of disease, drugs usually create problems in another part of the body. For example, while it is occasionally necessary to use an antibiotic to kill a potent bacterial strain, it will also wreak havoc on the intestinal flora. Similarly, all these medications place a burden on the liver, which has to keep de-toxifying the chemicals. Unfortunately, most people who have extreme cases of imbalance use many different medications, some of which add new symptoms.

The Fifth Cause

The last cause of disease Paracelsus cites is wrong physical habits which result in the "corruption of natural processes." He mentions overloading the stomach with excessive food, excessive drinking, and the use of certain condiments. For example, research has shown that a diet high in saturated fats leads to arteriosclerosis and other heart problems. Lack of exercise leads to poor circulation, conditions of overweight, and depression.

Paracelsus notes that many habits are psychologically caused. He speaks of association with the wrong people as a cause for excessive drinking. In order to discover why an individual tends to overindulge in food or drink, we must examine the cosmic level and the individual's horoscope for keys to understanding personal psychology.

HOW THIS BOOK IS ORGANIZED

Paracelsus focuses on the causes of disease; this book discusses therapies. As Paracelsus points out, a symptom may be due to a combination of causes. In the process of healing, a person can usually address the causes in any order, with work in one area leading to, and paving the way for, healing in another. And since all parts of healing are connected, many of the therapies discussed in this book address more than one cause of disease. However, they are grouped here according to their primary focus.

The first section includes therapies that seek to balance our magnetic fields (or the etheric body), and those that use the vibrations of various substances from nature. It includes such therapies as magnetic healing, healing with crystals and gems, music therapy, acupuncture, Reiki, and therapeutic touch.

The second section focuses on therapies that seek to balance our emotional, psychological, and spiritual states. Many of these focus on quieting the mind so that we can become attuned to inner peace. Other therapies focus on helping people experience emotions that they have repressed for a long time. These therapies address Paracelsus' second and third causes of disease. This section also includes chapters on two traditional systems of medicine— Traditional Chinese Medicine and Ayurvedic medicine—that tend to see physical imbalances as being caused by emotional and spiritual imbalances.

The third section focuses on correcting wrong physical habits and remedying the effects of introducing into the body various impurities, poisons, and harmful substances. The first chapter in this section covers methods of eliminating harmful substances from the body, and the rest of the section discusses various foods, herbs, and exercises that will help to re-balance the body.

The final chapter is a survey of diagnostic techniques that are used by many natural practitioners.

This book begins with some of the most esoteric therapies to emphasize the spiral of healing. Even though all parts of healing are connected, our society tends to blind us to all areas but the physical processes that can be described by scientists. It is my hope that by working in the opposite direction—from our need to be at one with cosmic energies, to how our spiritual, psychological, and emotional well-being affects our health; and finally, to the details of what substances are best for our bodies—this book will present healing in a more holistic way, as a spiral.

The spiral of healing is both a symbol and a physical current of energy. Symbolically, the spiral is an ancient, cross-cultural symbol of life and healing. Omnipresent in the old Goddess cultures, the spiral contains the infinite Mystery, which links our individual selves to the larger cosmos. This is different from a linear development suggested by a symbol such as a line or an arrow. Circular movements and symbols imply a matrix rather than a hierarchy. A *matrix* is a web of causes, all working together; a *hierarchy* implies a linear progression of causes where each factor is caused by the one below or above it. The spiral of healing balances the combination of planetary disturbances, psychic energies, emotional patterns, physical imbalances, and toxic substances that contribute to a state of disease or imbalance. Various therapies from Traditional Chinese Medicine to bodywork, to somatic techniques, form an interrelated web that helps to bring into balance our psyches and bodies. While some holistic healers and handbooks frequently ascribe a reductionist mode to their prescriptions—for this symptom, use this flower remedy or this herb; for this disease, think this thought—ultimately healing is a Mystery, and thinking of healing as a spiral can help us see that all levels of healing are interconnected.

The book's organization also emphasizes the literal spiral of healing—an energy current that goes from the non-physical body (often referred to as the etheric body) to the physical body, and back again. (In some esoteric literature, there are seven bodies that are referred to—the physical body, the etheric body, and five other "light" bodies; these are discussed in depth in the first chapter in the section on chakras.) For purposes of healing, we refer to the etheric body as the non-physical or spiritual body. Interestingly, the *caduceus* (symbol of the medical arts) also represents the physical spiral of healing. It is composed of a staff with wings at the top and two intertwining serpents curled around it. The two serpents symbolize two spirals, the left side representing feminine polarity, and the right side representing masculine polarity. The serpents' heads are at the top, suggesting that energy starts at the highest (non-physical) level and works down into the physical body.

Finally, I hope that by beginning with the therapies that address the universal forces acting upon us—the stars and global phenomena—this book will encourage all of us to think of our potential for healing as part of a universe that also has untold potential for healing if we give it our constant loving care.

PART I:
VIBRATIONAL
THERAPIES

CHAPTER 1:
VIBRATIONAL HEALING

Vibrational medicines tend to manipulate subtle energy fields by directing energy into the body rather than manipulating cells and organs through physical substances like foods and vitamin supplements, or through body adjustments or therapies. In this sense, they deal with what Paracelsus termed the "sidereal and astral" influences which act upon us. Since we are constantly getting bombarded by cosmic energies or forces, our electromagnetic fields continue to change and our nervous systems often become stressed. By utilizing the various forms of vibrational medicine, we can maintain our balance and learn to flow with the cosmic forces.

Vibrational healing is the oldest form of healing on the planet. Ancient tribes used sounds and tones, colors and crystals, and both the essence and aroma of flowers and plants, in their healing ceremonies. The present Holistic Health movement has reacquainted us with the principles of electromagnetic energy, which surrounds our subtle bodies. *Acupuncture*, the ancient Chinese form of healing, utilizes the meridian system which conducts electrical energy to the organs. Many of the *body therapies* now being practiced—Jin Shinn do, Shiatsu, polarity therapy, and Reiki—use this same energy.

Homeopathic medicine works with the vibrations of potent, natural materials. Remedies have little physical substance, but carry the vibrational quality of the substance in a pellet or globule which has a milk sugar base.

Colors emit vibrations, ranging from infrared to ultraviolet. *Sounds* also have vibrations; each note of the scale vibrates at a different frequency. *Crystals and gems* are part of the mineral kingdom; different crystals have their own unique vibration according to which crystal family they belong, how they are cut, and what size they are. *Flower essences and aromas* project vibrations, depending on the plants or flowers from which they are derived.

THE HUMAN ENERGY FIELD

Vibrational healing is based on the principle of light energy that surrounds the body. The presence of a luminous energy was first recorded by the Pythagoreans in 500 B.C. They believed that this light could produce various effects, including the cure of an illness. In the Middle Ages, Paracelsus and others, like the mathematician Leibnitz, perceived this luminous energy surrounding all beings. In the 1800s a physician named Mesmer wrote a dissertation on magnetism and suggested that an electromagnetic field existed. He was laughed at for his discoveries and attempts to use magnetism in healing.

In the mid 1800s Count Wilhelm Von Reichenbach studied the electromagnetic field which he called the "odic" force. Von Reichenbach found that the force in the human body produced a polarity similar to the one present in crystals along their major axes. He described the right side of the body as a positive pole and the left side as a negative pole.

In the 20th century, Kirlian photography has made people aware of the energy body. Through the use of electromagnetic apparatus, the film surface is charged, enabling the electrical energy or magnetic field surrounding the body to be photographed.

Many others have also been experimenting with the energy body. Dr. William Kilner, a medical doctor, reported on his studies of the Human Energy Field in which he used colored screens and filters. Kilner found that the aura differed among people depending on age, sex, mental ability, and health. He saw certain diseases as patches or irregularities in the aura.

Dr. Wilhelm Reich became interested in a universal energy that he called "orgone." He correlated the disturbances in the orgone flow in the body to both physiological and psychological symptoms. Reich observed pulsations from microorganisms with a special microscope and constructed a variety of physical apparatuses to study the orgone field. Later he integrated these with psychoanalytic techniques which worked to uncover unconscious blocks and then release negative emotional states through the use of orgone energy.

Most recently, studies were done at the University of California in Los Angeles by Dr. Valorie Hunt and colleagues. While studying the effects of a form of deep bodywork called rolfing on the human body, Dr. Hunt placed electrodes made of silver chloride on the skin and recorded the frequency of low millivoltage signals from the body. While she was doing this, Reverend Rosalyn Bruyere of the Healing Light Center in Glendale, California observed the auras of the rolfer and the person being rolfed. She reported the color, size, and movements of the chakras. The results of these experiments were analyzed; consistent wave forms and frequencies correlated specifically with the colors Reverend Bruyere reported.

THE SEVEN ENERGY BODIES

Not including our physical body, we have six other bodies that are not visible to the human eye, but whose energy can be detected. Each of these bodies has a center of energy called a *chakra* which is actually a whirling vortice of subtle energy. The concept of the seven chakras is delineated in both the Hindu and Tibetan systems, but many other healing systems, like traditional Native American healing, are aware of them. The chakras facilitate the flow of higher energy, via energetic channels, into the cellular structure of the physical body. There are seven major chakras; each is associated with a major nerve plexus and a major endocrine gland. They are in a vertical line, ascending from the base of the spine to the head. These channels follow the meridian system in Chinese medicine.

The chakras are connected to each other and to portions of the physical cellular structure through subtle energy channels known as *nadis*. The nadis parallel the nerves; there are about 72,000 nadis interwoven with the physical nervous system. The dysfunction of the chakras and nadis is associated with pathological changes in the nervous system.

The etheric body has the same structure as the physical body (including anatomical parts and organs) on which it is superimposed. The etheric body is composed of tiny energy lines that emit a bluish white light; it extends from 1/4 to 2 inches beyond the physical body. Within the etheric body is information that guides the growth of the physical structure of the body. It carries specifics on how the developing fetus is to unfold in utero and the data for growth and repair of the organism if disease occurs. The physical body is dependent on the etheric body for cellular guidance; if the etheric field becomes disturbed, physical disease follows.

Above the etheric body is the emotional body which is associated with feelings—longings, fears, and desires. The emotional body extends 1 to 3 inches beyond the physical body; its colors can vary from brilliant and bright to muddy and dark, depending on the clarity or confusion of the emotional state.

The next body is the mental body; it appears as a bright yellow light and extends 3 to 8 inches beyond the physical body. Through the mental body the self experiences intellect. Energetic forms known as "thought forms" originate in the mental body just as emotions originate in the emotional body. These "thought forms" have additional colors superimposed on them from the emotional level representing the individual emotion tied to the thought form.

Beyond the mental body are the next three bodies which are associated more with the spiritual world than with the physical. The astral or fourth body is like a higher emotional body. Its colors are similar to the emotional body but they are often infused with the rose light of love. A lot of interaction between people takes place on the astral level and colors may move back and forth when these interchanges are taking place.

The fifth body is a blueprint or template form for the etheric body. It extends from 1 1/2 to 2 feet beyond the body. When the etheric body is filled with disease, work on this level is needed. Healing with sound is particularly effective here; the throat chakra corresponds to the etheric template body.

The emotional level of the spiritual plane, the sixth body, is often referred to as the celestial body; it extends from 2 to 2 3/4 feet from the body. This is the level through which we experience spiritual ecstasy and unconditional love. The celestial body has appeared to many as a shimmering light with pastel colors predominant.

The seventh level is the causal body which extends from 2 1/2 to 3 1/2 feet from the body. This body is the mental body of the spiritual plane; it contains a grid structure of all the bodies and chakras and appears as a golden shimmering light.

THE SEVEN CHAKRAS AND THEIR MEANING

The first chakra, the *coccygeal center*, is related to physical vitality and will. When this chakra is blocked, the person lacks energy, may appear sickly, and does not make a strong impression in the world. When the first chakra is open, the individual can often energize those around him.

The second chakra, the *pubic and sacral center*, is related to giving and receiving sexual physical pleasure. If this center is blocked, there will be little sexual power and potency. When it is open, individuals are not afraid to share sexual energy or receive pleasure from it.

The *solar plexus*, located at the navel, is the third chakra. With the third chakra blocked, there is a loss of power and an inability to know what one can accomplish. When the solar plexus is open, individuals truly feel connected to the cosmos and to the unique place they have in it.

Fourth among the chakras and perhaps the most important is the *heart center*. If the heart center is blocked, there is an inability to feel love and affection. With an open heart center, the individual is able to love all human beings, animals, and other sentient creatures without expecting anything in return. Many cords are formed between individuals ("heart strings") when this chakra is open.

The *throat chakra* is the fifth chakra; it is related to our ability to speak out and voice our truth. If there is a blockage in the throat chakra, it may be due to holding back or not being comfortable enough in the world (third chakra) in order to express one's ideas and feelings. When this center is open, individuals speak out and express their deepest ideas and feelings.

The *third eye center* is the sixth chakra; it connects us with the ability to create and understand mental concepts. If there is a blockage in this chakra, the person may have confused mental concepts about the nature of reality; the concepts may also be negative. If, however, this chakric center is open, an individual is capable of visualizing ideas clearly.

The *crown center* is considered the seventh or last of the chakras; it is related to one's spiritual experience. If it is blocked, the individual does not have a connection to spirituality through personal experience. When it is open, there is a feeling of having experienced the state of transcendence which, in turn, creates a sense of personal faith and peace.

In order for an individual to function fully in the world, all the chakras need to be open with the "chi" flowing through each chakra. (A fuller discussion of "chi" exists in Chapter 5 on Traditional Chinese Medicine.) However, in many cases, there may be one or more chakras that are partially blocked and require some healing.

MAGNETIC HEALING

The earth's magnetic field is in constant flux; changes affect all living beings on the planet. Solar winds, shifts in the earth's core, and the presence of ferromagnetic substances in the earth's crust cause some of the variations. Several scientists have conjectured that the earth's magnetic field has degraded 50 percent over the last 500–1000 years. "Electric smog" from radios, televisions, computers, and other appliances have contributed to the degradation.

All living cells possess a positive electrical charge and a negative one that allow them to function in an orderly and healthy manner. As the electromagnetic charge wears down, the body attempts to send pulses of electromagnetic energy from the brain through the nervous system to recharge the cells and strengthen the field.

Magnetic field therapy seeks to help the body recharge its electric charges when the body is too depleted to do so itself. It utilizes the acupuncture meridians or energy channels, employing *bio-magnets* (tiny magnets placed in mattresses, pillows, and other devices). Its use has increased in recent years in both the treatment of body injuries such as sprains, broken bones, and burns, as well as in chronic conditions such as arthritis, degenerative joint conditions, and cancer. Through the use of electrical and magnetic therapies, healing time has decreased, and there have been many reversals of chronic conditions. Magnetic field therapy has been practiced longer in Japan than any other country, but, like acupuncture, is rapidly spreading to the Western world. As the earth's magnetic field decreases and the electrical smog increases, we will see more applications of magnetic field therapy.

Dr. Andrew Bassett, M.D., of Columbia University's Orthopedic Hospital and Presbyterian Medical Center, has achieved significant results using magnetic therapy for hip joint injuries and/or breaks. By utilizing electrically induced magnetic fields to cause regrowth of tissue, nerve, bone, and blood supply, 85 percent of his hip injury patients have been able to forego hip replacement therapy.

Dr. Kyoichi Nakagawa, M.D., one of the world's foremost experts on magnetism and its therapeutic effects on the human body, has been publishing reports in Japan since 1958 on magnetic field therapy. In both Japan and Korea, magnetic field products are licensed as medical devices. Dr. Nakagawa feels that the continual degradation of the Earth's magnetic field, combined with our electronic environment, is responsible for a broad range of symptoms which he labels the Magnetic Deficiency Syndrome. These symptoms include stiffness of the shoulders, back, and neck; low back pain; chest pains for no identifiable reason; headaches and heaviness of the head; dizziness and insomnia for unknown reasons; habitual constipation; and general fatigue.

Dr. Robert O. Becker, M.D., one of the American pioneers in healing with biomagnetic therapy, and author of *The Body Electric*, has achieved some incredible results in healing with biomagnetic therapy. He believes that electropollution may be contributing to Reye's syndrome, Lyme disease, Legionnaire's disease, and AIDS.

Dr. Buryl Payne, a physicist and psychologist who invented the first biofeedback instrument, has written two books on magnetic healing—*The Body Magnetic* and *Getting Started in Magnetic Healing*. According to Dr. Payne, sensitive research instruments have allowed scientists to document some of the ways magnetic fields affect living organisms. Specific factors that are involved include: increased blood flow with increased oxygen-carrying capacity; changes in migration of calcium ions which can either bring calcium ions to heal a broken bone in half the time, or can help move calcium away from arthritic joints; alteration of the *pH* (acid/alkaline) balance of various body fluids so that the capacity of sodium and potassium metabolism is increased in every cell; increase or decrease of hormone production from the endocrine glands; changes in enzyme activity and other biochemical processes.

Years of research and clinical tests have shown that the introduction of a magnetic field can provide the stimulation of the lymphatic system, as well as every cell in the body. The magnetic field does not itself heal; it merely aids the cells in creating an optimum environment in which the body can begin to heal itself.

There are many ways to implement magnetic field therapy. Magnetic sleep systems developed in Japan are among the most popular; magnets are placed in a mattress which is put on top of one's regular mattress. Initially some people feel worse because toxins may come to the surface when they first start using the mattress; others feel more energy immediately and can exist with fewer hours of sleep than before. I have used a magnetic pillow for a long time, which has helped to relax my neck muscles. I also use a magnetic car seat on my computer chair to deflect the radiation coming from the computer. In my own experience, individual magnets have been effective in healing burns as well as sprained ankles; they help increase the circulation and definitely speed up the healing process.

COLOR THERAPY

Color has been used since ancient times for producing certain psychological and emotional effects, and for healing and balancing the body. All humans, animals, and plants respond to differences of color and light throughout the cycle of a 24-hour day. Color is related to atmospheric density as well as light through its spectrum, ranging from infrared (high density) to ultraviolet (low density).

Color was first isolated by Sir Isaac Newton, who established the presence of seven basic colors in the spectrum by admitting sunlight through a prism. Each of the seven colors has its own wavelength. The variations of the wavelengths are the distinguishing characteristics of the color. When the wavelengths become very short, they become invisible to the human eye and are in the ultraviolet spectrum; when the wavelengths become very long, they are also invisible and are in the infrared spectrum. The essence of color healing consists of causing certain molecular reactions in the organism, or vital centers, through the medium of the rays.

In Tibet and other Oriental countries, color rays were used as a tool in meditation. Egyptian and Greek temples were painted various hues in order to have specific effects on their worshippers. In this century, Rudolf Steiner suggested the use of color and form as treatments for certain conditions. Dinshah P. Ghadali (1873–1966) established the Spectro-chrome Institute in Malaga, New Jersey where color therapy is combined with sound and rhythm and a color machine called a Spectro-chrome is utilized to beam the various colors onto portions of a patient's body. In England, the Hygeia studios in Gloucestershire use a color rhythm beamer developed by Theo Gimbel.

There are many forms of color healing. One can use the colors in foods for their nutritional benefits. Deep red foods such as beets, dulse, and cherries contain iron. Green leafy vegetables high in chlorophyll, which is the magnesium ion, also contain many essential minerals. Yellow foods such as squashes and peaches can have a laxative effect. Drinking water in colored jars that have been placed in the sunlight is another way of getting the benefits from that particular color.

One of the major ways to heal with colors is to use a lamp with color gels to focus any of the seven rays. There are two main kinds of ray treatment—general diffusion and local concentration.

In *general diffusion*, the light rays are focused on the body, especially the back, the region of the spine, and nervous system. This recharges the entire body and nervous system. The patient sits or lies down, stripped to the waist, and is immersed in light for thirty minutes. In *local concentration*, the light is focused only on the affected area. Light and color have a direct action on the protoplasm of the body and affect the speed of chemical reactions.

Other means of healing with color include placing colored glass in the windows of a room or in one's eyeglasses. Wearing clothes or gems of a particular color is a way of accenting that color in the aura. One of the best ways of color healing is through color breathing. Since air contains radiations from the Sun, stars, and planets, it contains all the colors of the spectrum. The color healer can practice deep rhythmic breathing with visualization of the rays. The first three rays—red, orange, and yellow, are magnetic and should be visualized as flowing up from the earth toward the solar plexus. The last three—blue, indigo, and violet, are electrical and are breathed in from the ether downwards. The green ray, the balancer of the spectrum, flows into the system horizontally.

Individual colors are chosen for their effects—red is used for blood poisoning, yellow to restore the nerves, green for vitality, blue for circulation, indigo for the muscles, violet for bone growth. Medicinal herbs and remedies often have the same color as the ailment. Iron, prescribed for anemia, is red; cathartics are yellow; disinfectants are green; and opiates are violet.

The meanings of the individual colors when used in healing are as follows:

Red (or **scarlet**) is a warm color and, therefore, a stimulant. It improves circulation and stimulates the nervous system, which energizes the senses of sight, smell, taste, hearing, and touch. It is also used in cases of anemia since it increases the hemoglobin in the blood. It causes expulsion of toxins through the skin and may bring in skin redness, itching, and pimples until the cleansing is complete. Red increases energy and aggressive tendencies. It works on the first chakra and can stimulate sexual energy.

Orange is related to calcium and is used to treat calcium deficiencies as well as to build bones. It is also a lung builder and respiratory stimulant. As an anti-spasmodic, it is helpful for cramps and spasms. As a digestive stimulant, it relieves flatulence in the digestive tract. It stimulates the thyroid and depresses the parathyroids. It also stimulates the mammary glands to increase milk production and increases eliminative discharges, bringing boils and abscesses to a head. Orange is an antidote to repression; it inspires self-confidence and positive thinking. Orange is related to the second chakra.

Yellow stimulates the motor nervous system, which energizes the muscles. It stimulates the production of bile, thus acting as a laxative. It also helps to increase hydrochloric acid and pancreatic *juices*. Yellow depresses the spleen and is helpful in expelling worms and parasites. Yellow is associated with the mental body and works well with the creation of thoughts. It is connected with the third chakra, the solar plexus center, and can raise vital energy.

Green has been considered the master healer; it is midway between the warm and cool end. It stimulates the *pituitary* (which in turn stimulates the other glands); dissolves blood clots; builds muscles, tissues, and skin, and destroys microorganisms like germs and bacteria. Green light provides the energy of the Sun in its most natural form, through plant energy known as chlorophyll, which is a source of magnesium and an excellent medicine for the heart. Green is connected with the fourth chakra, the heart.

Turquoise is an *excellent* tranquilizer; it is cooling and relaxing and helps headaches and swelling. It is also a skin tonic and rebuilds burned skin.

Blue is an antidote of red because of its cooling qualities. It relieves itching and irritation and is used for fevers, fast pulse, and pain, combating inflammatory conditions. Blue is also a stimulant to the pineal gland; it is a good antiseptic for the bleeding of the lungs, dysentery, jaundice, cysts, burns, and bruises. Blue has a soothing vibration and helps to heal the nervous system. It is connected to the fifth chakra, the throat chakra.

Indigo, a combination of blue and violet, is used to stimulate the parathyroids, depress the thyroid, purify the bloodstream, and treat convulsions and nervous ailments. It is also a mammary depressant. Indigo is related to the sixth chakra, the third eye, and is used to open up higher consciousness states.

Violet stimulates the spleen and promotes the production of white blood cells. It depresses the lymphatic glands and decreases muscular activity, including that of the heart. Violet helps to maintain the sodium/potassium balance in the body. It is used for bladder trouble, overactive kidneys, neuralgia, and nervous and mental disorders. Violet is a good remedy for diarrhea and induces deep, relaxing sleep. It is connected with the seventh or crown chakra and aids in the development of spiritual consciousness and psychic sensitivity.

Magenta, a combination of red and violet, is an important color for all heart disorders. It energizes the heart and stimulates the circulatory system and adrenal glands. It also helps to dissolve kidney stones as well as regulate blood pressure and arteries.

Various colors are found in the auras of individuals. The colors in the auras impart information concerning spiritual development as well as health and emotions. The major color indicating spiritual development seems to be stable, whereas the colors indicating physical health and emotional states appear to fluctuate. When the physical vitality is strong, the colors are clear. When the vitality is low, the colors may appear diluted; when fear, depression, or anxiety are present, they may be muddy.

The meanings of colors found in the aura are:

Red—Clear bright red shows moving anger. Dark red shows stagnant anger. Red-orange indicates sexual passion while rosy pink indicates pure unselfish love.

Orange—Bright clear orange shows health and vitality; deep orange—ambition.

Yellow—Golden yellow indicates high soul qualities; yellow in general shows intellectual prowess. An excess of yellow indicates an abundance of mental power.

Green—Green denotes nurturing, healing, and prosperity. Dark muddy green shows envy. An excess of green may show independence as well as healing ability.

Blue—Deep clear blue points to a pure spiritual feeling; bright blue shows sensitivity and sincerity. An excess of blue signifies an artistic, harmonious nature, and spiritual understanding.

Indigo—Indigo symbolizes moving toward a deeper connection with spirit.

Purple—Deep purple shows high spiritual attainment; lavender symbolizes spiritual consciousness.

White—Pure white emphasizes truth and purity.

Black—Black indicates forgetting, depression or invalidation, or thwarted ambition.

Grey—Grey shows depression and sadness.

Gold—Gold symbolizes a connection to the divine, and uplifted feelings.

Silver—Silver indicates deep communication.

MUSIC AND SOUND THERAPY

Sound as a healing modality is based upon providing tones to the body that it is lacking, or helping to remove tones that are causing blockages or inhibiting certain physiological processes. The healing qualities of music have been recognized from the earliest times. Paracelsus used music to cure a variety of mental, emotional, and physical ailments. He prescribed special compositions for certain illnesses in accordance with the law of vibrations.

Throughout history, sounds in nature have evoked a wide variety of emotions in humans—the howl of a coyote in the mountains, the soothing sound of a stream bed, the laughter of children playing. Many traditional cultures have used drumming to help connect the spiritual dimensions with the physical one. Other cultures have used special instruments for making sound, such as Tibetan bells or Peruvian whistles, to help us release our energies from mundane earthbound concerns and move into another dimension.

Until recently, it was thought that sound was perceived through the ear. But new developments in the study of vibrations have shown us that we perceive sound through the entire body. Because sound is vibration, there are many vibrations that we sense which are either too low or too high for our ears to hear. That is why so-called "deaf" people hear so much; they are hearing other frequencies.

Sound is a slower vibration of light. The Hindus believed the Universe was created from sound; they called the first sound *Nada Brahma*. (Brahma is one of the three central Gods in Hinduism, and *Brahman* comes from the Sanskrit root *bri* which means "to grow" but also "to praise"; everything that is growing and alive is Brahma. Nada Brahma means not only God is sound but Creation, the cosmos, the world is also sound.) Vibrations from sound create light and darkness as well as color. There are exactly 44 octaves between middle C at 256 Hz and the color of deep red 44 octaves higher at 4.6×10^{15} Hz. Each sound has a color equivalency; some of these colors can be seen by the human eye while others are in the infrared or ultraviolet spectrum.

Each chakra also has a tone connected to it; middle C is the root chakra. However, these tones may only correspond to our chakras when we are in a state of harmony. In nonharmonious states, the color and tone relationships may be off.

Dr. Hans Jenny, a Swiss scientist, spent many years observing and photographing the effects of sound upon inorganic matter. He put water and other liquids, plastics, and dust on steel plates and then vibrated them with various frequencies. Once they were exposed to sound waves, these inanimate blobs began to move and formed new shapes. Dr. Jenny named his work

Cymatics (from the Greek *cyma* which means wave), and he wrote about the relationship between harmonics and harmonious patterns.

The body itself is composed of many vibrational patterns which work together as one whole. Certain muscle groups and organs have a particular resonance; larger ones have a deeper resonance and smaller ones a less deep resonance because their wavelengths are shorter. The immune system, nervous system, blood system, respiratory system, all have different vibrations. Specific pieces of music and certain tones resonate to the different organs, muscles, and body systems. African drumming music with a strong beat will vibrate the denser tissues and may help loosen the patterns that have become entrenched there. Gregorian chants may vibrate the more subtle tissues and add tones that may be missing.

In highly stressed individuals, the voice and body patterns will have a higher pitch. This is also true of those with sensitive nervous systems. A more relaxed individual will generally speak slower and in a lower pitch.

After World War I, Margaret Anderton, a musician and nurse, conducted some experiments among wounded Canadian soldiers. She found that it was most beneficial to have someone administer music for any form of war neurosis, which was predominantly mental, but for orthopedic cases or paralysis, it was most beneficial if the wounded person produced the music themselves. Anderton reported that memories were brought back to men suffering from amnesia, and that paralyzed muscles were restored.

Dr. Paul Nordoff, an American composer, and Clive Robbins, a special educator working with handicapped children, used music therapy with autistic, Down's Syndrome, and brain-damaged children. The therapy which they developed has been utilized at a hospital in London. When working with individual children, the therapist improvises vocally and at the piano to try to present the children with an experience of the mood they are feeling—frustration, rage, or anxiety. The children are then encouraged to respond on percussion instruments, on the piano, or with their own voice.

Alfred A. Tomatis, a French physician, specialist in otolaryngology and author of *The Conscious Ear*, has been studying the functions of the human ear and the importance of listening to particular sounds. Tomatis believes that there are two kinds of sound—sounds that fatigue the listener and sounds that "charge" the listener. He was called to a Benedictine monastery where seventy of the ninety monks were exhausted, unable to work, and eating foods they had never desired. Upon discovering that the new abbot had eliminated 6 to 8 hours of Gregorian chanting from the monks' daily schedule, Tomatis started them singing again and also hooked up each monk to head phones with baroque music. Within nine months, all but two of the monks were vigorously working and feeling rested with less sleep. Tomatis believes that the high frequencies in this music supplies essential electric charges to the brain.

One of the pioneers in using sound for healing is Dr. Peter Guy Manners, an English osteopath. After studying Hans Jenny's work on cymatics, Manners developed a cymatics instrument composed of a portable computer and a sound generator. The harmonics from the cymatics instrument are a composite of five different frequencies that Dr. Manners found most effective for healing the body. These sounds are electronically created; some of them are scientifically created and some are determined through radionics or radiesthesia. Using devices such as pendulums, which seem to swing back and forth in response to this energy, radionic practitioners have been able to develop frequencies for every part of the body. The cymatics instrument has frequencies for every organ in the body and for specific diseases. There are also frequencies for emotional and mental problems. Some imbalances treated with cymatics are asthma, anemia, colitis, diabetes, heart disease, and sciatica.

In the 1930s Dr. Royal Rife discovered frequencies for eliminating cancer and later uncovered the frequencies which specifically destroy herpes, polio, spinal meningitis, tetanus, influenza, and a number of other diseases. Rife found that every cell has its own vibratory frequency, and every cell within a specific organ system has a similar vibratory frequency. If there was a disease of a particular group of cells, he could find the frequency that would remove the diseased cells. The specific frequency was known as the *Mortal Oscillatory Rate* or M.O.R. Rife also worked with polarity techniques which were different from frequency applications. Applying energy to induce changes in the polarity of the electrical charge of certain tissues prevents most viruses and bacteria from reproducing. This technique is often used as a follow-up to frequency therapy sessions.

Although many scientists and doctors confirmed Rife's discovery of the cancer virus and his method of working to eliminate cancer, they later turned against him when his work became known. Many of the records were stolen from Rife's lab, his virus microscopes were vandalized, and Dr. Milbank Johnson, who ran Rife's clinic, was found to be poisoned during a tonsillectomy. Today there is one Rife microscope at the Smithsonian Institute and many people have reproduced Rife machines in the United States, Canada, and Germany. Those who are using Rife machines for healing today are aware that in order to be free of disease, the individual has to continue a regimen of cleansing and eating pure foods, as well as looking at any psychological patterns that have caused the disease.

Another frequency-based healing modality that utilizes harmonics is Barbara Hero's *Lambdoma frequencies*; the Lambdoma is a mathematical table by Pythagoras of ratios based on overtones. Barbara Hero, an artist and mathematician, has created a series of tapes designed to balance the chakras based on these frequencies.

Sharry Edwards, a healer from Athens, Ohio, has been doing healing work through sound therapy based both on the voice and on frequencies. Edwards hears the signature sound, the sound made by every living thing, and then she is able to reproduce that sound. At her institute, Sound Health Alternatives, she teaches others to find the signature sound, as well as healing many people with various ailments who are not responding to other therapies. Edwards refers to her work as Bio-Acoustics; she has developed computer programs to detect the frequencies that are missing in individuals. She then exposes the individual to those frequencies. The brain waves and pulse are monitored before and after the exposure to the frequencies.

One example of her work was with a young boy in West Virginia whose heart was racing at 150 beats per minute and he was in line for a heart transplant. After hooking him up to the computer, she diagnosed that it was a metabolic problem and his doctor agreed. He was given certain frequencies and his diet was also adjusted; his heart began to beat at a normal rate within a few weeks.

Another individual with a heart problem was found, through the computer, to be lacking taurine, an amino acid that helps build the heart. He was given the frequency of taurine for seven weeks; this was done by listening to sounds on a small machine that resembled a tape recorder. He listened to the sounds as much as possible, which change the brain wave pattern if it's missing a frequency. Within seven weeks, his heart was normal.

Edwards and her colleagues are researching many diseases including various types of cancers. They have also observed some interesting patterns about obesity. Overweight people appear to have some poison or toxin that they aren't aware of because the fat is insulating the body from that poison. Once the toxin or poison is removed, their weight drops. Edwards teaches many week-long seminars to train practitioners to do this type of work.

A modern form of music therapy is toning, originated by Laurel Keyes. Since the tone of a person's voice is indicative of the state of health, the sound of the voice may encourage negativity. A tone might carry hostility and resentment, so the individual constantly gets negative reactions from people.

Toning involves a cleansing of the whole being and a tuning of the higher self so one is aware of what one is really feeling. To tone, one stands with eyes closed, relaxing the jaws and letting the sounds come out. One may do toning along with certain exercises like yoga or stretching. Toning stimulates the energy flow in the body.

Toning can also be done in groups for healing. One of the objectives of toning groups is to send healing to those in need. The effects have been quite dramatic, and there are many cases of those who have been healed through toning. A nurse who had been a diabetic with uremic poisoning and multiple sclerosis came to see Laurel Keyes and her sister. Laurel and her sister toned for her for 20 minutes. She experienced a breakthrough in which she sobbed and began to understand what was going on in her body. As she began to tone for herself, the uremic condition cleared up, her vision improved, and the multiple sclerosis was halted.

Dr. Randall McClellan, author of *The Healing Forces of Music*, created a system for balancing the chakras using the human voice. He developed a harmonic series with overtones for the chakras; each chakra resonates to a note which is a certain mathematical distance above the chakra below it.

Kay Gardner, musician and author of *Sounding the Inner Landscape: Music as Medicine*, uses a system of harmonically related notes for the chakras. Gardner uses C for the root chakra, D for the second chakra, E for the third chakra, F sharp for the heart chakra, G for the throat chakra, A for the third eye chakra, and B flat for the crown chakra.

Another healing use of harmonics involves the way in which the brain resonates with these sounds. Many individuals are aware of vibrations in their head when they create vocal harmonics. Karlheinz Stockhausen, a German composer and mystic, was the first one to compose music for overtone singers. Stockhausen observed changes in the skulls of the singers he trained to create vocal harmonics. He theorized that the changes may not just be related to the bones of the cranium, but may have affected the brain as well. Stockhausen has trained several overtone singers including Jill Purce, a British overtone singer who teaches many sound healing workshops in the United States.

The uses of sound and music for healing are growing daily. One of the influences of this movement is to bring chanting and toning to more people as a way of balancing energy and maintaining health.

HEALING WITH CRYSTALS AND GEMS

Since the formulation of the Gaia hypothesis in the 1970s, we are learning that the human body cannot be separated from the body of the earth. What is used in the earth to heal herself can also be used to heal us. Crystals and gemstones have been used in many ancient cultures for thousands of years. *Crystals* are found deep in the earth's surface; they carry electromagnetic energy and amplify the energy field when placed in the same room or on the body during a massage. Many believe the larger purpose of crystals is to maintain the balance between the electrical energies surrounding the earth and the magnetic energies between the poles. *Gems* are also mined from the earth; they have been used both externally and internally for healing.

Crystals come in different shapes and sizes as well as different colors. Like radio transmitters, they have the power to amplify our energies, positive or negative. *Generator crystals* are clear single quartz crystals that are used to channel and ground healing energy; they allow light to come through them. Generator crystals are often held above the chakras or placed on them directly during a crystal healing. *Crystal clusters* consist of several single terminated crystals with a common base; they can be placed in areas where one wants to create a stronger healing vibration, or to cleanse old and negative energy from an area. Smaller crystals and stones can be purified by being put on clusters for a few hours. There are many potent types of crystals such as double terminated crystals, tabular crystals, window crystals, phantom crystals, and crystal balls.

For individual healing, a crystal layout is the form most commonly used. In this process, the healer or the healee chooses one or more particular crystals for each chakra. These crystals match the color and vibration of the corresponding chakra. Often larger crystals or several smaller ones are placed where there is the strongest blockage. The healer then works on each chakra in turn, clearing the energy and re-balancing. When this is completed, the crystals are removed and purified. Usually they are put in a bath of sea salt and water to soak overnight. Sometimes, after the bath, they are placed out in the sun for thirty minutes and wiped dry with a soft cloth. They can also be cleansed by they purifying smoke of cedar, sage, or sweetgrass.

Gemstones were used in Egypt for healing purposes. The *Ebers Papyrus* recommends the use of certain astringent substances such as lapis lazuli as ingredients for eye salves. In India, Ayurvedic physicians used the ashes of gemstones, which had been pulverized, in the preparation of special medicines. In Roman times, Pliny compiled material on gems, categorizing them by color, constitution, and which diseases they could cure. A distinction was made between the talismanic quality of stones for the cure and prevention of disease, and the medicinal use of them as mineral substances. In the former case, they were worn on the person, while in the latter, they were ground in water or some other liquid.

As talismans, stones were engraved with a symbol or figure at a certain time of the day and month when various planetary forces were operative. This process gave maximum benefit to the wearer. The Star of David, the pyramid, the ankh, and the cross were commonly used symbols since they carried a certain vibratory character in addition to the stone's vibration. Rulers of countries wore crowns of precious stones to enable them to rule wisely, and rings on various fingers to channel particular energies into their lives. Belly dancers wore rubies and deep red stones in their navel to stimulate sexual interest in their viewers. Necklaces hung in the area of the chest stimulated heart chakra points for greater love and compassion, while stones worn on earlobes were intended to stimulate reflex points.

Gemstones are still used internally as gem essences. The stone is placed in water and some alcohol such as vodka or brandy and put out in the sun for a few days. This liquid then contains the vibration of the particular stone and is used as a mother tincture for making bottles of the gem essence. Various gem essences are recommended for both physical and emotional conditions.

Color was an important part of the use of the particular stone. Red stones, like the ruby, garnet, carnelian, and bloodstone were considered remedies for hemorrhages and inflammatory diseases. Yellow stones such as citrine were prescribed for bilious disorders, jaundice, and other diseases of the liver. Stones of green hue relieved diseases of the eye due to the beneficial influence exerted by this color upon sight. Lapis lazuli, sapphire, and other blue stones were believed to heal the nervous system. Purple stones such as amethyst were said to counteract the effects of intoxicating beverages.

Following is a list of some of the most important crystals and gems associated with the seven chakras:

First Chakra—red, also black

Garnet—Garnets are small blood-colored stones. They impart passion, energy, and courage. When placed over the womb, garnets are used to improve fertility and ease menstrual cramps and irregularities. They help cleanse the blood and improve circulation. Garnets are also used on the third eye (sixth chakra) to facilitate past life recall.

Coral—Coral consists of reefs growing on the floor of warm seas. Dark red coral is a stimulant and tonic to the bloodstream. It is also used as a remedy for depression and as a heart energizer.

Ruby—Rubies aid in the circulation of the blood and in cleansing infection from the blood. They are also beneficial in dissolving blood clots if used in conjunction with a prism. Rubies strengthen the adrenal glands and have been used to stanch the flow of blood when ground up with water and used as a paste.

Bloodstone—Bloodstone is a deep green stone interspersed with bright splotches of red jasper. It has been associated with mysticism in India where much of it is mined. Bloodstone is used to stanch hemorrhages and to prevent nosebleeds. It is a good stone to use in balancing energy because it contains both green and red—yin and yang.

Smoky quartz—Smoky quartz contains the most amount of light found in a dark stone. It helps to channel energy from the crown chakra to the first chakra and ground it on the physical plane. Smoky quartz works to dissolve toxins in the body as well as repelling negative emotions; it can be placed on any area where there is pain or blockage.

Black obsidian—Obsidian comes from lava which has cooled quickly. Although it is black, you can see through it easily. It is good for those who feel cut off from the source of light as well as those who need physical grounding. Black obsidian acts as a mirror to magnify fears, insecurities, and egocentric attitudes. In crystal healings, black obsidian is placed on the navel or groin to help pull higher energies into the body. Black obsidian balls are powerful meditation pieces.

Second Chakra—orange

Carnelian—Carnelian is a red-orange agate which generates warmth and may help to dispel confusion and absentmindedness. It is useful for infertility or impotency when placed around the navel and pelvic area. It works to clear the reproductive organs of any blockages and can also be placed over the second chakra for sluggish digestion.

Third Chakra—yellow

Citrine—Citrine is a yellow quartz crystal which derives its color from iron oxide. It helps one access personal power and brings about a sense of self-approval. Citrine aids in relaxing digestive organs, helping constipation, and also with relaxing the diaphragm so one can breathe better. It is excellent for mental activities; it aids concentration and can help the mind let go of responsibilities and worries.

Topaz—Topaz was associated with the ancient Egyptian Sun god Ra, the giver of life and fertility. Topaz can impart inner strength because of its color and clarity. It is used in treating tension headaches since it helps bring about the relaxation of cells within the head. It also helps with depression and insomnia.

Fourth Chakra—green and pink

Malachite—Malachite is one of the basic ores of copper and is often found along with azurite. Malachite has the power to dredge up emotional pain; when it is released, the wearer may feel joyful and light-hearted. Because of its deep green color, malachite is very grounding. I often wear malachite beads the day after flying because they help me to ground and be part of the earth again. In ancient Egypt, malachite was used for cosmetic purposes; when ground up and mixed with water, it was painted on the eyelids.

Green jade—Jade is considered to be one of the most precious stones in China and Japan. The Chinese believe that it provides a link between the spiritual and the worldly. Green jade brings in the subtleties of nature; it is balancing for the whole body and carries a vibration of love and forgiveness. Jade can also draw impurities from the body; it is used over swollen glands in the neck. A small piece of green jade is a wonderful meditation stone.

Green aventurine—Green aventurine is a quartz with a pure green ray. It is good for dissolving emotions that are causing constriction in the heart area and may be used in conjunction with malachite, which brings emotions to the surface. Aventurine has the power to soften those who have difficulty expressing their feelings. Green aventurine can be carried or worn during times of stress since it brings healing to all areas of the body.

Emerald—Emerald is a stone that has been used for centuries. Its green color is effective in grounding one on the earth plane, in quieting the emotions, and in balancing the aura. Physically, it strengthens the heart and spine, helps alleviate problems associated with diabetes, and strengthens the adrenals. The main use of emeralds in ancient times was in bathing the eyes with water infused from steeping the stones for several hours.

Watermelon tourmaline—Watermelon tourmaline is green underneath and pink on top, both of the colors associated with the heart chakra. The Rosicrucians and alchemists called tourmaline *christus stone*, which symbolized the ascent of matter (green) to sublime love (pink). Watermelon tourmaline is used in crystal healings when individuals really want to open their heart and be vulnerable to their deepest feelings. It is also used to negotiate with someone who is rigid and intractable, in which case it is good to have the stone in one's pocket or close at hand.

Rose quartz—Rose quartz derives its pink tint from titanium. Its soft pink color comforts and heals any wounds the heart has accumulated. It is used in crystal healings for those just beginning to open up to their feelings as well as for those who need the comfort of the Divine Mother. Rose quartz is also used for skeptics who have not yet opened their spiritual consciousness.

Fifth Chakra—blue and blue-green

Turquoise—Turquoise has always been considered a sacred stone by the Native Americans, who use it in jewelry and ritual objects. Turquoise loses color when its wearer is ill or in danger; it turns a dull yellow when worn by a person with liver problems. Turquoise increases one's vibratory rate and enhances healing powers. It has been used to treat eye problems as well as ailments of an inflammatory or feverish nature.

Azurite—Azurite is a deep blue indigo stone which is often found in combination with malachite. Azurite enables us to speak about our deepest feelings and problems when placed at the throat chakra. Azurites are also used to heal the eyes; when the eyes are tired from driving or computer work, place a small azurite on each eye near the corner and lie down and rest. After a half hour, the eyes will be rejuvenated. These stones also bring insight as to the causes of diseased conditions.

Sixth Chakra—blue-violet

Lapis Lazuli—Lapis Lazuli is a deep blue stone mixed with white calcite containing specks of gold pyrite. Lapis has a strong spiritual *vibration*; it is said to be one of the stones in the breastplate of the High Priest as well as being the stone on which Moses inscribed the ten commandments. In ancient Egypt, it was known as the stone of the Gods; the gold flecks symbolized the stars in the night sky and were regarded as touchstones for truth. Lapis is often placed on the third eye to facilitate visualization and attunement to higher spiritual teachings. Lapis is useful in meditation; placing a piece of flat lapis at the crown center will help the energies to rise.

Sapphire—Sapphire, like lapis, is a sacred gemstone. Ayurvedic physicians use it to treat mental illness as well as rheumatism and colic. It can be placed on the eyes to relax them; it is also used to overcome fever and the effects of poisons in the body.

Fluorite—Fluorite comes in pyramids, octahedrons (two pyramids joined together at the base) and clusters; it is mostly blue, purple, white, or gold, though there are some pink and green fluorites. The six-pointed octahedron helps to create a sharp focus and relaxes the mind when it is tired. It should be placed on the third eye. Fluorite allows one to see the wisdom behind outer world appearances. It is often used in treating certain types of mental illness and disturbances in brain wave frequencies. Fluorite increases the electrical charge of the brain cell which brings more energy into the brain. In crystal healings, fluorite is usually placed on the sixth chakra or third eye center; when it is removed, it is often unusually warm, indicating the amount of activity that it has stimulated.

Seventh Chakra—violet or purple

Amethyst—Amethyst is a powerful protective stone; it has the ability to dispel all negative influences when placed in a room. Amethyst is also a very relaxing stone; it can be put under one's pillow during sleep, especially if there are nightmares or bad dreams. As a meditation stone, it is often placed on the third eye or crown; deep transformation is possible through using the amethyst.

Amethyst is also helpful for migraines and, when placed in boiling water, the liquid is used to cleanse the skin.

Sugilite (Luvulite)—Sugilite is a new stone on the planet, having been discovered in the 1970s. It has a deep purple color, deeper than fluorite or amethyst. It is an excellent stone to be used by super sensitive souls who tend to take on the vibrations and emotions of others. Like amethyst, it should be used in meditation, on the third eye center or crown, and in rituals. Sugilite is cleansing to the lymph system when placed on the groin or near the lymph glands. There is not much sugilite on the planet at this time, but probably more will be available as we need it.

Opal—Opals vary in color from milky white to greenish yellow to fiery red; there are also black opals. Like the seventh chakra, they contain a lot of light. Opals hold a large amount of water and some air; they change color when the wearer is very emotional. Opals are considered mystical stones and tend to enhance memory; when used in meditation, they are often placed on the third eye center.

Clear quartz crystals—Clear quartz crystals contain the full spectrum of color of the seven rays. They help to bring more light and color into the aura and can balance out any blockages in the physical or emotional bodies. Since they vary greatly in shape and size, particular ones will be chosen to accompany other crystals in a crystal healing.

FLOWER REMEDIES

Flower remedies or flower essences are subtle remedies derived from wildflowers. They use the healing power of the flowers to create within us a condition in which we are more emotionally balanced and less prone to disease.

Essences are prepared from a mother tincture which is made by infusing flowers with water out in the sunshine. The Sun acts as a catalyst to draw out the aura or etheric body of the flower. That is, the water contains very little of the flower's physical substance, but its energy permeates the water. (This is similar to the principle of homeopathic medicine. See Chapter 3 on homeopathic medicine for more information.) This liquid is then preserved with alcohol (usually brandy) and used as the mother tincture from which stock bottles are made. Remedies may be taken internally through the mouth in a dropper or placed in a bath where they penetrate the whole body. Several remedies may be taken at once in combination.

Flower remedies penetrate the circulatory system first, entering the bloodstream, and then the nervous system, where they are transmitted through electromagnetic energy to the meridians and in turn to the subtle bodies and the chakras.

There are several different ways of determining which flower remedies should be utilized at a certain time period. An interview and consultation should take into account the patient's emotional history, noting any fears, anxieties, or personality dysfunctions that exist. Some practitioners use a pendulum or dowsing rod to determine which remedies are best for the person. (see Conclusion). Others use muscle testing.

The first flower essences were developed by Dr. Edward Bach, an English physician who worked in bacteriology in a London hospital. After experimenting with vaccines of toxic substances to boost the immune system, he turned to homeopathy. Bach developed homeopathic *nosodes* (potentized extractions of disease matter, tissue, or discharges) for the seven types of bacteria associated with chronic illness. He discovered that patients carrying each of the seven types of intestinal bacterial pathogens displayed particular personality characteristics. This led him to further research on emotional factors and personality types contributing to illness. Since he did not like administering nosodes prepared from disease-producing agents, he went out to look for flowers whose essence would work with emotional patterns. Bach stated, "Providential means have placed in nature the prevention and cure of disease by means of divinely enriched herbs and plants and trees. They have been given the power to heal all types of illness and suffering."

Dr. Bach felt that illness was a reflection of disharmony between the personality and the higher self; this disharmony causes dysfunctional energetic patterns in the subtle bodies. The flower essences realign emotional patterns so that patients increased their physical vitality and thus could fight their disease. Patients suffering from an unknown fear would be given aspen; those from a known fear or phobia, mimulus; those who were in shock, a combination of remedies known as "Rescue Remedy" containing star-of-Bethlehem, rock rose for terror and panic, impatiens for mental stress and tension, cherry plum for desperation, and clematis for faraway, out-of-the-body feelings.

Following Dr. Bach's footsteps, an American healer named Richard Katz began experimenting with flower remedies made in the Sierras and at Mount Shasta in California. Many of the essences he developed work on removing blockages involving sexuality, intimacy in relationships, spiritual transformations, and achieving higher states of conscious awareness. Katz developed the Flower Essence Society with his wife, Patricia Kaminski. Purposes of the Flower Essence Society include utilizing the healing properties of plants, establishing a network of communication with practitioners around the world who are utilizing flower remedies, researching new remedies, and conducting classes and retreats involving the essences. The Flower Essence Society has several kits including many of their essences. They also have a number of publications available including *Flower Essence Repertory*, which lists different emotions and categorizes all the remedies (including the Bach remedies) under their appropriate emotions.

Machaelle Small Wright, working with the devic energies, developed a nature research center in the foothills of the Blue Ridge Mountains in Virginia called Perelandra. Here she made the Perelandra garden and rose essences described in her book *Flower Essences*.

AROMATHERAPY

Similar to crystals which are found in the earth and flower remedies that are extracted from flowers, aromas, or essential oils are derived from plants and flowers. Unlike using the leaves or roots of a plant as Herbology does, Aromatherapy extracts only the oil. (In *Herbology*, the physical part of the herb is used to make a tea, tincture, or salve; it affects the physical cells of the body.) Over the years, with the pollution of the air, water, and soil, plant fibers are weaker in color and nutritionally less potent. However, when the oil is removed, the same strong vital force is there. The oil carries the life force of the plant much as a homeopathic remedy carries the life force of the substance from which it is derived.

It is this essence or vital force that is able to work with the electromagnetic field and help to balance it.

The term *aromatherapy* was coined about 50 years ago by René Maurice Gottefosse, a French chemist. Aromatic oils are used in foods, toiletries, and medicines. In foods, they are used as natural flavorings, such as oil of lemon and orange. In cosmetics, they are incorporated in perfumes and in toothpaste flavorings. In medicines, they are used as therapeutic agents; for example, clove oil for toothache, peppermint for indigestion, and eucalyptus oil for respiratory problems.

Essential oils are odorous and readily evaporate in the open air. They are completely soluble in alcohol and ether, and partially soluble in water. They are present in tiny droplets in a large number of plants and are responsible for the scent of flowers and herbs. They move from one part of the plant to another according to the time of day and season.

Essences are extracted by distillation. This involves placing the plant material in a vat and passing steam through it. The essence escapes along with water and other substances. The distillate is cooled, and the essence is then separated from the water.

Heat, light, air, and moisture have a damaging effect on essential oils. They should be kept in dark airtight bottles and in cool, dry conditions.

Essential oils are taken from herbs and plants. Certain flowers emit a strong fragrance or scent as part of their reproductive process. Once they become impregnated, the fragrance ceases.

Essences have a long history. They were used by the Egyptians who put them in cosmetics, massage oils, and medicines. Priests were the first to use the aromatics, and later they were also used by physicians. The aromatics used in Egypt included myrrh, frankincense, cedarwood, origanum, bitter almond, spikenard, henna, juniper, coriander, calamus, and other indigenous plants. Cedarwood oil was also used in the process of mummification.

The ancient Hebrews used essential oils in many of their religious rituals. Women were given a 12-month purification with myrrh oil. There are many references to essential oils in the Bible. In Exodus, God gave Moses a "holy anointing oil" (Exodus 30:22-25). Among the gifts of the Wise Men to the Christ child were frankincense and myrrh.

Learning from the Egyptians, the Greeks attributed the origin of aromatics to the Goddesses and Gods and used various oils in their perfumes as well as to anoint specific parts of the body. The Greek physicians recognized the difference between stimulating and sedative properties in the essences. The Romans were even more lavish in their use of perfumes than the Greeks. The knowledge of distillation, however, remained forgotten since Egyptian times. An Arabian physician known as Avicenna is credited with this invention in the tenth century. Avicenna first used the rose and later distilled other essences.

The Chinese used aromatics with their acupuncture, and many essences are written about in the Hindu Ayurvedas. Sandalwood was one that was used as an incense and an unguent or salve. In the Middle Ages, the herbalists and alchemists worked with essential oils and were familiar with the process of distillation.

In modern times, research has been carried out in regard to the antiseptic properties of essences. This research has been conducted primarily by chemists and pharmacists. René Gottefosse was a chemist interested in the cosmetic use of essences. He soon gathered enough information to convince him that many essential oils have even greater antiseptic properties than some of the antiseptic chemicals that were in use. Then, one of Gottefosse's hands was badly burned as a result of a small explosion in his laboratory. He immersed it in lavender oil and found that the burn healed at a phenomenal rate with no infection or scarring.

A colleague of Gottefosse named Godissart set up an aromatherapy clinic in Los Angeles. He was successful in achieving cures for skin cancer, gangrene, osteomalacia (softening of the bones as a result of an imbalance in calcium and phosphorous metabolism), facial ulcers, and bites from black widow spiders using lavender oil.

Gottefosse published his first book *Aromatherapie* in 1928. Meanwhile, another Frenchman, a medical doctor named Jean Valnet, began to use essences in his treatments. He used them during the war in treating battle wounds and in many pathological conditions. Dr. Valnet administered the oils orally—a few drops in a little sugar.

Marguerite Maury, author of *Marguerite Maury's Guide to Aromatherapy: The Secret of Life and Youth*, and a French biochemist, treated the whole person—mind, body, and psyche—with essential oils. She dissolved the oils in vegetable oil and used them in massage treatments so that they absorbed through the tissues of the body; in this way, they worked on internal problems as well. She found that bergamot, chamomile, and lavender stimulated the production of white blood cells when rubbed on the skin or inhaled.

Italy has also produced some researchers in the field. Doctors Gatti and Cajola working in the 1920s and 1930s, realized the scope of therapy with essential oils. Paolo Roveti of Milan worked with citrus oils indigenous to Italy—bergamot, lemon, and orange—and also demonstrated clinically the benefit of certain essences in states of anxiety and depression.

There are many methods of getting essential oils into the bloodstream other than by taking them internally. Essential oils penetrate the skin. An essential oil placed on the foot will be distributed to every cell in the body within 21 minutes.

Essential oils are aromatic and many benefits can be obtained simply by inhaling them. Diffusing essential oils into a room is an excellent system of air purification. They increase the ozone and negative ions in the house, which inhibit bacterial growth; they help to remove metallic particles and toxins from the air, and they destroy odors from mold and animals and fill the air with a fresh herbal scent.

Essential oils have the ability to carry oxygen and nutrients through the cell walls and can therefore help to bolster the immune system and prevent disease. They have a very high frequency and help to build up the body's frequency which drops when colds and flus set in, thereby compromising the immune system.

CHAPTER 2:
VIBRATIONAL BODYWORK

There are many therapies that use physical contact to affect the body's electromagnetic energies or to influence the energy body. Oriental therapies work with chi; chi is the vital life force that flows through the body. Some Western therapies seek to balance electromagnetic currents. Other therapies help to cleanse the chakras so that emotional or psychic depletions are removed. In psychic surgery, a Latin American technique, a healer works with the etheric body to gain access to the interior of the physical body.

ACUPUNCTURE AND ACUPRESSURE

The system of *meridians* or lines of force running through the body derives from ancient Oriental healing modalities. These meridians are used in acupuncture, acupressure, shiatsu massage, Jin Shin jitsu, and Jin Shin do. Each meridian is connected to one of the vital organs; there is a liver meridian and the points on this meridian send electromagnetic energy to the liver. If the liver is congested or stagnant, or if there is too much heat in the liver, stimulating these points can help to balance the situation. Acupuncture utilizes needles which are inserted under the skin into certain points on particular meridians, depending upon the condition. The meridians and points are determined by the acupuncturist after a diagnosis is made through the pulses and the tongue. (See Chapter 5 on Traditional Chinese Medicine for a thorough discussion.) Acupressure utilizes these same points with finger pressure; the points are often referred to as *tsubos*. Acupuncture is used for chronic conditions, for diseases of the internal organs, and as an anesthetic. Both acupuncture and acupressure are utilized for colds and flus, headaches and backaches, menstrual cramps, and boosting the energy level. With acupressure, pressure is generally applied for 5 seconds, and then released for 5 seconds. If a point is sore, it indicates a blockage of chi. By stimulating that point, either with finger pressure or a needle, the chi is released and the soreness usually disappears.

JIN SHIN

Jin Shin Jyutsu was developed by Jiro Murai in Japan at the beginning of the 20th century. He treated many people but taught the art to only six people, one of whom is still alive—Mary Burmeister, who lives in Arizona. Early students of Mary's have introduced Jin Shin under the titles of Jin Shin do and Jin Shin acupressure. Jin Shin works on synchronizing pulses and utilizes eight other meridians besides the twelve organ meridians used in acupuncture. The twelve organ meridians are like rivers or streams, and the eight extra meridians are like reservoirs or lakes. When the river becomes full, it spills into the reservoir; when deficient, it draws from it, offering a system of checks and balances. The chi or vital energy flows through these channels; when the flow becomes stagnant, an imbalance results creating stress or tension, and eventually illness. Jin Shin releases this stagnation by using these eight additional meridians. Instead of the heavier pressures applied in acupressure and shiatsu, Jin Shin uses a light pressure and works through the clothing. When necessary, Jin Shin can avoid physical contact by placing the hands over a particular area to remove pain. As the energies are unblocked and made to flow, the body can heal itself.

POLARITY THERAPY

Polarity therapy was developed by Dr. Randolph Stone; it is based on balancing energy circuits and fields within the body. Dr. Stone set up a system of positive and negative magnetic polarities based on anatomical relationships within the body. He also utilized the elements—earth, air, fire, and water, and designed charts for the energy flow of each element in the body.

A treatment of polarity therapy involves subtle finger pressure on various areas of the body. The polarity therapist usually starts out by standing behind the head of the person and later moves to the feet. As one area is worked on, the attention is then brought to another area which is energetically related; in this way, a balancing effect is achieved. Gentle manipulations are sometimes included.

REFLEXOLOGY

Reflexology works with the electromagnetic currents in the body; these currents can be accessed through the reflex points in the feet which connect to other parts of the body.

The principles behind reflexology or zone therapy were known in ancient China and used by some American Indian tribes. Reflexology generally works with the feet; whenever certain points in the feet are sore, it indicates that the corresponding organ is out of balance. In reflexology, the body is divided longitudinally into ten zones. The hands have the same reflexes as the feet and can be used instead of the feet. There are also cross reflexes linking shoulder and hip, elbow and knee, hands and feet. The pressure applied to the reflex points varies according to the practitioner and the person being treated. By massaging these points periodically, there is improved circulation, elimination of toxins, and greater flow of the chi.

HANDS ON HEALING

Throughout the ages, people have been healed simply through touch, through the energy of love that is channeled through the hands. Though anyone is capable of doing this type of healing, certain individuals are particularly gifted and can feel the heat coming through their hands when they are working on another person's body. Studying the human energy field and being able to read the aura and the energy in the chakras is a great help in knowing where to focus the healing energy, and in visualizing the removal of blocks and toxins in specific areas. An excellent book to use is *Hands of Light: A Guide to Healing Through the Human Energy Field* by Barbara Ann Brennan. Hands on healing by a group of people (often termed "laying on of hands") can be particularly potent since all are working at the same electromagnetic field.

REIKI

Reiki (universal life energy) is an ancient form of hands on healing that was developed in Japan by a Japanese monk named Mikao Usui in the 19th century. The Reiki practitioner acts as a channel for chi energy or universal life force by using the hands as electrodes. With the practitioner channeling the energy, the client's own innate wisdom draws as much Reiki as is needed. Utilizing various patterns of energy flows in the body, the Reiki treatment is able to provide specific energy to the source of the problem, or unblock the vital force in a specific organ.

Reiki classes are centered around "empowerments" or "attunements" whereby the teacher opens the student's energy centers and aligns them with Reiki. Each class consists of a theoretical framework for Reiki, its history, and how and when to use it; there is also a lot of practice and discussion. There are three levels of Reiki classes; each one deepens the student's proficiency in Reiki. The Level I class enables the student to give "hands on" treatments. The Level II class focuses on absent treatments and more emotional issues, while Level III enables a student to become a teacher.

THERAPEUTIC TOUCH

Therapeutic touch, developed by Dolores Krieger, Ph.D., Professor of Nursing at New York University, is another way of transmitting energy through the laying on of hands. Therapeutic touch uses sweeping motions to cleanse the aura of the body prior to working on specific areas. This technique involves four phases: the first is to center oneself to become a conduit for the universal life force; the second is to assess the bioenergetic field of the other person by passing one's hands through the front and back of the field; the third is to mobilize the areas in the patient's energy field that are blocked, deficient, or out of balance; and the fourth is to direct the healer's energy to help the patient re-pattern which includes unblocking, filling holes, and balancing.

Therapeutic touch brings relaxation and pain relief; it has helped acute conditions like burns and headaches as well as more chronic ones such as arthritis. Many nurses are using this technique to work with those in the process of dying; the touch is soothing and brings energy to the heart area where it is particularly needed.

PSYCHIC SURGERY

In *psychic surgery*, the energy body is disconnected from the physical body so that the tissues become an amorphous jellylike mass. The diseased tissues are removed and afterwards the two bodies are reconnected. The surgery itself takes only a few minutes; the patient does not feel anything at all. The healer penetrates the etheric body through the hands; no instruments are used. There is blood surrounding the area penetrated, which is washed off after the diseased part of the organ is removed.

Psychic surgery has become very popular in both the Philippines and Brazil. I experienced psychic surgery with a Filipino healer who had traveled to the United States. After penetrating my skin with his hands, a process that was immediate and in which I felt nothing, he removed a small piece of tissue from my colon. There was quite a bit of blood which was removed by a nurse who was assisting. He then balanced my energy centers and prayed over me. The whole process took about seven minutes. I felt very balanced and energized after the surgery.

The healer who worked on me spoke no English so I could not tell him where I was experiencing difficulty in my body, yet he went to the spot immediately. I learned from another Filipino man who was traveling with the healer, that this particular healer belonged to a certain family who resided on one of the islands and they were all trained in this technique. They were very spiritual people who were not involved with the intellect. I watched this particular healer work on several other people and was amazed at how quickly he worked and how accurate he was in his knowledge of those areas of the body that needed healing.

CHAPTER 3:
HOMEOPATHY

Homeopathy affects the body's electromagnetic field through the use of remedies based on natural substances. These remedies have only a minute amount of the physical substance, but strongly carry the energy (or electromagnetic information) of the substance.

According to George Vithoulkas, a contemporary practitioner of homeopathy and author of many books on the subject, the aspect of the vital force which establishes balance in states of disease is known as the "defense mechanism." Samuel Hahnemann, the 19th-century German physician who developed the science of homeopathy, theorized that when disease occurs, the first disturbance occurs in the dynamic electromagnetic field of the body which then brings into play the "defense mechanism." Hahnemann believed that a therapeutic agent could act directly upon the electrodynamic field and thereby strengthen the defense mechanism.

Hahnemann's research consisted of finding a substance whose frequency had a similar resonance to the individual's own and could thus affect the electromagnetic field. He sought substances that would produce similar symptoms. He believed that any substance which could produce a totality of symptoms in a healthy human being could cure those symptoms in a sick human being. This cure had to affect all levels of being—the mental/spiritual, the emotional/psychic, and the physical.

The "law of similars" is basic to homeopathic practice; it is utilized in immunizations and vaccines against diseases like smallpox, diphtheria, and typhoid, as well as in allergy treatment where small doses of allergens are used to create an antibody response. In the 4th century B.C., Hippocrates worked with the law of similars. He stated, "Through the like, disease is produced, and through the application of the like it is cured."

The usage of micro-doses is also basic to homeopathy. Hahnemann believed that a person's inherent healing powers were strong enough so that only a small stimulus was needed to catalyze the healing process. After many years of experimentation, Hahnemann found a method of diluting substances that kept the toxic properties at a minimum. This method called *potentization* is a process of successive dilution. If the medicine is soluble, one part is diluted in 10 parts water or alcohol, and the mixture is mixed vigorously. If it is insoluble, it is finely ground or triturated in the same proportions with powdered lactose (milk sugar). One part of the diluted medicine is diluted again in the same manner, and the process is repeated until the desired strength is obtained. A remedy that has been diluted fewer times has a lower potency. It has been found that the more a substance is potentized, the deeper and longer it acts, and the fewer number of doses are needed in treatment.

Potentization has stirred controversy among certain scientists who believe that if a substance is potentized to a very high dose, there will be very little of the physical remedy left. Dana Ullman, however, reports in his book *Homeopathy: Medicine for the 21st Century* that evidence for the efficacy of small doses was given in *Science News*. A study engaged in by chemists noted that when they shook coupled molecules of nitric oxide, the units did not weaken and break into parts, but developed stronger molecular buds. The homeopathic process of dilution and succession (shaking) therefore creates super-strong molecules.

In prescribing a certain homeopathic medicine, a patient's symptoms are noted. Symptoms of most importance concern the patient's relationship to the environment, food, sleep, sex, and habit patterns rather than the clinical details of the physical symptoms. Hahnemann derived his system of remedies for specific symptoms through "provings." *Provings* consist of the systematic procedure of testing substances on healthy human beings in order to elucidate that the symptoms reflect the action of the substance. The remedy is tried on a healthy person in toxic as well as diluted doses. Symptoms on all three levels are noted, as well as those symptoms that have disappeared from the patient after a cure has been produced.

Homeopathic remedies are catalogued in books known as *Materia Medicas*, which are compilations of these drug provings that associate certain symptom pictures as well as physical and emotional characteristics with various substances. There are also *Repertories* available—books which list certain symptoms and the remedies known to heal them. Most well-known of the *Repertories* is that of Dr. J. T. Kent, which has a word index including all parts of the body and all types of conditions that affect these parts.

After the administration of a homeopathic remedy, symptoms on the deeper levels improve while those on more external, superficial levels may temporarily get worse. The principles of the homeopathic healing process were first observed by Constantine Hering, a German homeopath who emigrated to the U.S. in the 1830s. These principles are known as *Hering's Law,* or the "Law of Direction of Cure." Hering observed that "the body seeks to externalize disease," to dislodge it from more serious internal levels to more external levels. As an example, people with asthma may find their lungs getting better, but they may develop a skin rash.

The first aspect of Hering's Law states that healing progresses from the mental and emotional levels and the vital organs to the external parts like the skin and the extremities. Eventually, even the superficial symptoms are alleviated. A cure is in progress if psychological symptoms lessen and physiological symptoms increase. As a guide to this law, George Vithoulkas has provided the following list of symptoms. Symptoms from each level, in order of depth, are as follows:

Physical: brain, heart, endocrine, liver, lung, kidney, bone, muscle, skin

Emotional: suicide, apathy, sadness, anguish, phobias, anxiety, irritability

Mental: confusion, delirium, paranoia, delusions, lethargy, dullness lack of concentration, forgetfulness, absentmindedness

The second aspect of Hering's Law states that healing progresses from the upper to the lower parts of the body. Pains in the neck and chest area might appear in the legs, but the person would be considered to be on the mend.

The third aspect says that symptoms appear and disappear in the reverse of their original order of appearance. It has been observed by homeopathic doctors that patients experience symptoms from past conditions, especially in dealing with chronic illnesses. The symptoms may be from illnesses ranging from six months to many years. In homeopathy, when symptoms become worse, it is referred to as a "healing crisis." This is often necessary to achieve a complete healing on a deep level. While one is undergoing the healing crisis, one's vital force is becoming stronger.

These laws are not always observed in each person's healing process. Symptoms may also proceed upward in the body. The important thing is that the individual begins to feel stronger, that old symptoms disappear, and that a change in the psychological makeup of the individual is apparent.

Depending on the symptoms present, the homeopath may choose to administer a second dose of the same remedy or another remedy. Sometimes one remedy clears out certain symptoms and paves the way for another remedy.

ADMINISTERING REMEDIES

Depending on the form of the remedy, one dose would consist of one drop of the liquid, about ten of the tiny little granules, or three to four of the larger pellets. It is best not to touch the remedy, but instead to pour it onto or under the tongue. It is also important not to take water or food with the remedy for 15–20 minutes before or after administering it.

Certain substances have been found to antidote homeopathic remedies, particularly coffee and products containing camphor (cosmetics, lip balm, nail polish, Vick's™, Noxema™). These substances do not always antidote the remedy, but if the original symptoms return after drinking coffee or using products with camphor, it is best to repeat the remedy.

CHOOSING THE CORRECT REMEDY

In order to choose the correct homeopathic remedy, it is important to make careful observations of the person and to note all her/his physical and psychological symptoms. Physical symptoms include general strength and energy level, muscular coordination, restlessness, sleep patterns, response to temperature changes, thirst and appetite, food cravings, color of skin and tongue, pulse, and type of body odor. Psychological symptoms include mood changes, state of mind, desire to be with others or left alone, neatness and orderliness, self-image, and efficiency in completing projects.

After studying a person's symptoms, a homeopath attempts to find a remedy that matches the person's totality of symptoms. Certain symptom patterns are identified with medicines that have healed them; for example, the "Nux Vomica" type, the "Phosphorus" type. Treatment may consist of a repetition of the same remedy in a different potency or another remedy.

In Europe, certain homeopathic practitioners utilize several remedies for different sets of symptoms. This practice is known as *Pluralism*; there is no formal research comparing it with classical homeopathy.

In addition to the "constitutional remedy," there are also remedies for many acute conditions like burns, bee stings, colds, coughs, sprains, etc. It is possible for the layperson to utilize these remedies with the help of a book, such as Stephen Cummings' and Dana Ullman's *Everybody's Guide to Homeopathic Medicines* or Dr. Maesimund Panos' *Homeopathic Medicine at Home.*

COMMON REMEDIES

There are certain common homeopathic remedies that are included in homeopathic first-aid kits and should be available in each household. A short description of these follows.

Aconitum Napellus (monkshood)—Aconite is useful in the early stages of inflammation or fever, or the first stage of a cold. Typical is hot, red skin, strong thirst, sometimes a throbbing headache. There is anxiety and restlessness, acute panic, and fear.

Allium Cepa (red onion)—This remedy is good for colds, respiratory allergies, sneezing, runny nose and eyes, stuffed nose, hoarseness and beginning laryngitis, neuralgic pains, and sinus headaches.

Apis Mellifica (honeybee)—Apis relieves insect bites, bee stings, hives, and other injuries that involve stinging, burning pain.

Arnica Montana (leopard's bane)—Arnica is used for bruises, falls, injuries, pain after dental extractions, soreness of muscles, joint sprains, and shock from injuries.

Arsenicum Album (arsenic)—Arsenicum is used for burning pains, especially of the throat, stomach, or eyes. Discharge of the nose or diarrhea often burns and irritates the skin. Heat and warm drinks are helpful. There is often restlessness and fear as well as severe weakness and exhaustion.

Belladonna (deadly nightshade)—Belladonna is helpful in the acute early stages of inflammatory illnesses characterized by high fever and severe pain that begin suddenly and end abruptly. Intense heat, redness, throbbing, and swelling are key symptoms. Fevers, sore throats, earaches, and skin eruptions are treated with belladonna.

Bryonia Alba (wild hops)—The person requiring bryonia is irritable, easily angered, and often wants to be left alone. There may be a dry, hard cough, headaches, a strong thirst for large amounts of liquid, and often constipation with dry, hard stools. Motion aggravates any of these conditions.

Calcerea Phosphorica (phosphate of lime)—Calc Phos aids the healing of bones and is good for fractures, teething, pains in bones and joints, colic in babies, and promoting milk in breast-feeding mothers.

Cantharis (Spanish fly)—Cantharis alleviates pain from burns and scalds; it is also helpful for painful, burning urination, and cystitis.

Carbo Vegetabilis (vegetable charcoal)—Carbo Veg is an important remedy for stomach gas. There is often heartburn, regurgitation of food, and burning in the stomach. It is also good for one whose energy is low after a serious illness.

Chamomilla (German chamomile)—Chamomile is soothing to the nervous system; it is good for sleeplessness, nervous conditions, and pain. It is often given to irritable, fussy children, especially during teething.

Ferrum Phosphoricum (phosphate of iron)—Ferrum Phos is a great remedy in the beginning stages of inflammatory conditions such as colds, flu, rheumatism, or bronchitis. It is good for those suffering from allergies and anemia.

Gelsemium (yellow jasmine)—Gelsemium is often recommended in damp weather. The person requiring this remedy often feels heavy and tired and mentally sluggish. They often experience chills running up and down the body. Anxiety and anticipation may bring on these symptoms.

Hypericum Perfoliatum (St. John's wort)—This is a good remedy for injuries to the nerves. It is also helpful for injuries to the fingertips, nails, toes, and tailbone, as well as in treating severe concussions and eye injuries. It has also been found to be helpful in treating depression.

Ignatia Amara (St. Ignatius bean)—Conditions calling for ignatia are those that are precipitated by emotional stress, such as grief, anger, or disappointment. It is used for conditions of the nervous system that are a result of strong emotions and overstimulation.

Ipecacuanha (ipecac root)—Ipecac relieves nausea with or without vomiting; it also helps to stop nosebleeds or bleeding from any part of the body.

Ledum Palustre (marsh tea)—Ledum is the chief remedy for puncture wounds, stings, and bites.

Magnesia Phosphorica (phosphate of magnesium)—Mag Phos eases any pains or cramps, such as menstrual cramps, leg cramps, or colic. It is good for severe nervous conditions and sleeplessness.

Mercurius Vivus (quicksilver)—Mercury is required during acute conditions where there is inflammation of the skin and mucous membranes along with pus formation and open sores; urinary infections; and skin infections such as boils and herpes.

Nux Vomica (poison nut)—Nux Vomica is used after overindulgence in food, alcohol and drugs. It is a good remedy for the liver and works well for intestinal flus.

Pulsatilla (windflower)—Pulsatilla is a remedy that is often used for menstrual problems—delayed menstruation, PMS, and menopausal symptoms. Those needing pulsatilla tend to be sensitive, vulnerable, moody, and desire attention. It is also a good remedy for certain cases of allergies, digestive upsets, ear infections, and colds.

Rhus Toxicodendron (poison ivy)—Rhus Tox is helpful for inflamed skin blisters from poison ivy and oak, chickenpox, and herpes. It also works well for sore muscle and joint pains that are relieved by motion.

Ruta Graveolus (rue)—Ruta is helpful for injured, bruised bones and for sprains after arnica is used. It is also beneficial for sciatica and headaches due to eyestrain.

Sulphur—Sulphur is used most often for chronic conditions. Sometimes these conditions involve dry, scaly skin; sometimes constipation with dry, hard stools. There is usually a great deal of thirst, flushes of heat, and improvement with fresh air.

CELL SALTS OR TISSUE SALTS

The biochemic system of medicine was developed by Dr. W. H. Scheussler of Germany in the late 1800s. Dr. Scheussler explained disease and body imbalance as a result of the molecular disturbance in certain cell salts or trace minerals in the body. He found twelve of these to be the most abundant constituents of cremated human remains. He therefore theorized that an adequate supply of all twelve was necessary to prevent disease.

Although Dr. Scheussler's explanations are overly simplistic, the twelve cell salts, which are homeopathically prepared, have been extremely useful in balancing conditions in the body. Dr. Hahnemann and his colleagues have included provings of these in the *Materia Medica*. The cell salts are obtainable in low potencies such as 3x, 6x, 12x, and 30x, but they are also available in higher potencies.

Since each person's chemistry and metabolism are so different, the proportion of tissue salts varies in each of our bodies. We may have an inherent tendency to lack one or more of the salts, and at various times in our life we may develop deficiencies of any of the salts. We also may have more of the tissue salts.

Some of the salts seem to be more useful than others, as proved by the testing of individuals. For example, the sodium salts are rarely needed because most people have too much sodium in their bodies. On the other hand, the potassium salts are called for a great deal.

Descriptions of the twelve salts follow.

Kali Phos (potassium phosphate)—Kali Phos is found in all the tissues and fluids of the body, particularly the brain and nerve cells. It is a great nutrient for the nerves. A deficiency of Kali Phos may produce irritability, timidity, fearfulness, and sleeplessness. It is a good remedy for headaches, depressions, insomnia, and conditions of nervous origin.

Nat Sulph (sodium sulphate)—The principal function of this salt is to regulate intracellular fluids in the body by eliminating excess water. It is important to the proper functioning of the kidneys and bladder.

Kali Mur (potassium chloride)—This salt unites with albumin, forming fibrin, which is found in every tissue of the body with the exception of the bones. Fibrin helps cells retain their shape. Kali Mur is helpful in treating any respiratory problem, such as colds, hay fever, allergies, bronchitis, sore throats, and tonsillitis. It is often taken in a high dose at the first sign of a cold or flu.

Calc Fl (calcium fluoride)—Calc Fl appears in the surface of the bones, the enamel of the teeth, and the elastic fibers of the muscle tissues. Its deficiency causes these tissues to lose their elasticity. It is useful in treating diseases of the teeth, bones, hardening of the arteries, and conditions such as arthritis and rheumatism.

Mag Phos (magnesium phosphate)—Mag Phos is anti-spasmodic in that its work relates to the nerves. A deficiency of this salt causes the body to contract, producing spasms and cramps. The contraction puts pressure on the sensory nerves, which give rise to sharp, shooting pains. Mag Phos is good for cramps associated with menstruation, muscle spasms, epileptic conditions, and heart conditions. Though a larger dose of magnesium is required for all the above conditions, Mag Phos can be helpful as well.

Kali Sulph (potassium sulphate)—Kali Sulph carries oxygen to the cells of the skin and distributes oil in the body, which aids in perspiration and the elimination of body poisons. Kali Sulph is excellent in the treatment of acne and other skin conditions, including dandruff.

Nat Phos (sodium phosphate)—Nat Phos maintains the acid/alkaline balance in the blood. Lack of this salt may produce a yellow coating on the tongue. Nat Phos is helpful in relieving stomach acid and in treating ulcers.

Calc Sulph (calcium sulphate)—Calc Sulph is a blood purifier which builds the epithelial tissue in the body. It is effective in the healing processes of the bones, joints, and teeth and is used in elimination problems such as constipation.

Silica (silicon dioxide)—Silica is present in the blood, bile, skin, hair, and nails. It is also found in connective tissue, bones, nerve sheaths, and mucous membranes. In proper amounts it gives fingernails, hair, and teeth a glossy appearance. It needs to be used with the appropriate amount of calcium to be effective.

Calc Phos (calcium phosphate)—Calc Phos is a constituent of the bone tissue. The body requires large amounts when it is growing or recovering from fractures. It also plays an important role in the clotting mechanism of the blood. Lack of Calc Phos causes skeletal problems such as rickets, curvature of the spine, and swollen or painful joints. Calc Phos is helpful for teething and all problems with teeth and bone where calcium is required.

Nat Mur (sodium chloride or table salt)—The most useful of the sodium salts, Nat Mur is found in every cell and fluid; one of its most important roles is to maintain the proper degree of moisture within the body. A deficiency of this salt may cause an imbalance of water in the body, and the individual may appear very bloated and sometimes may suffer the opposite condition of excessive dryness. It is useful in watery blisters, insect bites and stings where it is applied externally in a solution. It is also helpful for dryness of tear ducts, sneezing, and post-nasal drip.

Ferrum Phos (iron phosphate)—Found in the blood, Ferrum Phos is an essential component of hemoglobin, which carries oxygen to all parts of the body. It is the most frequently needed of all the tissue salts because most diseases start with inflammation of one kind or another. Ferrum Phos is essential for red blood cells and its lack can cause anemia. Due to the difficulty of assimilation of iron, Ferrum Phos in all potencies is a most helpful remedy.

PART II:
THERAPIES
FOR THE MIND,
EMOTIONS,
AND SPIRIT

CHAPTER 4:
MENTAL AND
SPIRITUAL THERAPIES

Paracelsus stated that the second and third causes of disease were spiritual, emotional, and psychological problems. Spiritual and psychological healing are closely related, since spiritual progress usually comes only after we have quieted our minds and emotions sufficiently to feel our own oneness with the Universe. Modern research has confirmed the connection that Paracelsus drew between the mind and body. We know that not only can long-term states like depression affect the immune system, but so can day-to-day emotions like anger, sadness, frustration, love, and joy. We have also learned that altering our emotional states can improve the body's ability to fight infection. For example, Norman Cousins showed how laughter can change the course of an illness; he healed himself by learning to transform his own emotional states through laughter.

The therapies discussed in this section seek to transform our emotional states to more health-promoting states, or to give us greater control over our minds. In order to work with our emotions and transform our emotional states, we have to learn to acknowledge and access all of our feelings, whether they be positive or negative. Acknowledging our frustrations, our anxieties, and our fears actually boosts the number of natural killer cells in the bloodstream. If we hold on to these emotions over too long a time period, these same cells can become depleted. A reaction of grief to the death of a close friend can boost the immune system whereas a reaction of long-term depression can deplete it. Working with these various emotional states and their effects on the immune system is known as *psychoneuroimmunology* (PNI). Psychoneuroimmunology studies the effects of the nerve fibers forming direct contacts with the cells of the immune system. Research has shown that hormones and neurotransmitters influence the activities of the immune system, and that products of the immune system can influence the brain.

In certain psychiatric disorders, there are hormonal changes that affect the immune system; sudden fright or fear causes an outpouring of adrenaline which also alters the immune system. A patient's will to live enhances the immune system while feelings of loneliness deplete it.

Faith in the healing process is a strong element in building the immune system. Many doctors write of the *placebo effect*, the fact that about one third of patients will show improvement if they simply believe they are taking an effective medicine, even if the pill they are taking has no active ingredient. Tumors have grown smaller, cancerous cells have disappeared, symptoms have changed overnight when patients believed the substance would heal them. Dr. Howard Brody of Michigan State University feels that a positive placebo response occurs when three factors are present: the meaning of the illness is altered for the patient in a positive way, the patient is supported by a caring group, and the patient's sense of control over the illness is enhanced. In all traditional societies, any type of physical healing procedure is accompanied by prayer or ritual—usually both. Ritual brings in the higher forces and affirms that there is more to wellness than just manipulating the physical body or imbibing some physical substance. Prayer gives the patient hope and faith that some change will occur; it strengthens the belief system, helping one to becoming whole again.

Many healers and medical practitioners realize how much the emotions are involved with the healing process. In his books, Dr. Bernie Siegel deals with the importance of communicating openly with patients and dispensing love and nurturing, especially to those who have been branded with the label "terminal illness." He speaks of learning what the patient's belief system is and having the physician share his belief system as well. In 1978, Dr. Siegel started ECaP (Exceptional Cancer Patients), a form of individual and group therapy based on "carefrontation." He uses guided imagery, meditation, hypnosis, and dream work in his therapy. Dr. Carl and Stephanie Simonton explored these ideas further in their work with cancer. The Simontons explained how the imbalance known as cancer often manifests after some trauma in one's life such as the death of a family member, separation from an important relationship, or loss of a job. The Simontons have worked with breaking up old emotional patterns and changes in lifestyle to accommodate new ways of thinking. Louise Hay, in her early book, *Heal Your Body*, made associations between different emotional states and particular organs, such as problems with the throat or a sluggish thyroid being related to not speaking one's truth or frequent headaches often experienced by those who are heads of large organizations or businesses. Other healers such as Barbara Brennan have related emotional imbalances to block-ages in various chakras as well as organs; a throat or thyroid problem might then originate from the fifth chakra, the throat chakra, and this chakra might become clear if we speak up and don't hold back our feelings.

There are many ways to enhance immune system response—starting with simple relaxation and meditation techniques, visualization, biofeedback, and hypnosis, as well as working with process-oriented techniques of transper-sonal psychology and past life regression.

RELAXATION

Relaxation involves withdrawing the mind and the body from external stimu-lation in order to reach deeper levels of consciousness. The aim of relaxation is to let go of tensions in the body, anxieties and worries in the mind, and if possible, enter a light trance where the brain operates at a slower frequency, referred to as alpha waves. With the brain operating at a slower frequency, one becomes more centered and is able to restore vital energy more readily.

Brain waves have been designated in four categories—delta, theta, alpha, and beta. These terms were coined by Hans Berger in 1924 who was studying EEG readings as an attempt to understand how telepathic impressions are received. Berger assigned these Greek letters to the particular wave forms and spectra of electrical activity recorded by the electroencephalograph. Alpha waves (8–12 cycles per second) were researched by psychologist Joe Kamiya in the 1950s. (See the section in this chapter on Biofeedback.) Theta waves (4–7 cycles per second) are present during drowsiness and sleep, and are associated with daydreaming, imagery, and creative visualization. Elmer and Alice Green at the Menninger Foundation have trained people to augment theta activity for the enhancement of creativity and to catalyze paranormal experiences. Theta treatments have also been used for sleep disorders. Delta states register below 4 cycles per second. Yogis have been tracked in delta during samadhi, a state of spiritual enlightenment. We all reach theta and delta states during sleep, but we have not yet learned how to stay awake in these states. Beta waves have a frequency of 40 cycles per second and are associated with learning processes. Beta wave training has been used to relieve learning disabilities.

In his book, *The Relaxation Response*, Dr. Herbert Benson was the first to discuss the purposes of relaxation in medicine and healing. Progressive relax-ation therapy consists of exercises done with different sets of muscles; part of the technique consists of making the patient aware of tension being held in particular muscle groups. Beginning with the dominant hand and forearm and working gradually along the body, select one group of muscles and tense them as forcefully as possible, holding the tension for about 10 seconds, and then releasing it for 30 seconds. When you relax the muscle group, try to make it even more relaxed than it was before.

Relaxation is necessary for meditation and visualization to occur.

MEDITATION

Meditation is a tool for training the mind to develop greater calm, and using that state of calmness to bring insights into our own experience. It's a way of slowing down in order to get in touch with who we really are, and the rhythmic flow of the universe. It enables us to do our work with a stronger awareness and consciousness.

There are many techniques that are useful in entering a meditative state. A common one is to focus on the incoming and outgoing breath while sitting in a still position. If the mind wanders, bring it back to the breath, focusing on the ebb and the flow. Sometimes gazing on an image such as a candle is helpful in quieting the mind. Another method which is used in many Hindu practices is the use of a *mantra*, the repetition of a certain sound or series of sounds. In meditating, one needs to keep the body still and to remain detached from thoughts, sensations, and emotions. Meditation improves concentration, and in time, can lead to experiences that are deeply spiritual.

Physical benefits of meditation have been well documented. In his book, *The Relaxation Response*, Dr. Benson showed that meditation tends to lower or normalize blood pressure, pulse rate, and the levels of stress hormones in the blood. It also produces changes in brain wave patterns. In 1976, a research study was conducted by Gurucharan Singh Khalsa, founder of Boston's Kundalini Research Institute. The study was conducted at the Veterans Administration Hospital in La Jolla, California and showed that regular yoga and meditation increased blood levels of three immune system hormones by 100 percent. Jon Kabat Zinn started a Stress Reduction clinic at the University of Massachusetts Medical Center in 1979 in order to help people access their inner resources for healing and operate more effectively in the world while coping with stress. In the clinic, meditation and yoga were taught in a simple way with other techniques of relaxation and scanning the body. Patients experienced less tension in their bodies as a result, and often uncovered emotional problems that had been contributing to their illness.

In 1980 psychologist Alberto Villoldo of San Francisco State College showed that meditation and visualization improved white blood cell response and the efficiency of hormone response to a standard test of physical stress—immersing one arm in ice water. Those trained in meditation withstood the pain—better than those who did not meditate.

VISUALIZATION

The ability of the mind to bring forth positive images and to visualize the body as healed is very powerful. Visualization therapy was developed by Dr. Carl Simonton through his work and treatment of cancer patients. Dr. Simonton, working together with his wife Stephanie, had patients mentally picture their disease to see how their bodies were interacting with the treatment so they could hasten the recovery process. For example, he would have them visualize an army of healthy cells overcoming the cancer cells. Jeanne Achterberg, with her husband Frank Lawlis, expanded the work of the Simontons, incorporating various types of imagery. Jeanne has written a book in the history and use of images in healing called *Imagery in Healing: Shamanism and Modern Medicine.*

Visualization is so effective because the body does not distinguish between a mental and a physical experience. A cancer patient can visualize himself performing like an athlete, and in time, this can become a reality. Drawing or painting can enhance the process of visualization. The more concrete the images are drawn on the mental plane, the greater chance they have of becoming reality on the physical plane.

Charles Garfield, a psychologist at the University of California Medical Center in San Francisco, noted that similar techniques were used by cancer survivors and by Soviet and Eastern European athletes who were successful in the Olympics.

HYPNOSIS

Hypnosis is a state of consciousness where the critical factor of the mind, occurring mostly in the brain's left hemisphere, is put to sleep, allowing suggestions to be accepted and repressed memories recalled. Hypnosis has been important in treating many conditions of physical imbalance or disease, especially those stemming from emotional traumas and those that have a psychoneurological basis.

The first book to mention hypnosis is a book called *Neurypnology or the Rationale of Nervous Sleep* by Dr. James Braid (1795–1860), a Scottish physician. Dr. Braid suggested that the combined state of physical relaxation and altered conscious awareness entered into by patients should be called *hypnosis* (from the Greek word *hypnos* meaning "sleep"). In 1829, a French surgeon, Dr. Cloquet, performed a successful mastectomy without the use of other anesthetics on a 64-year-old hypnotized woman. During the surgery, as a malignant tumor was cut out by incisions made from the armpit to the inner side of the breast, her heart rate and respiration remained normal and she felt no pain.

Modern hypnosis is referred to as *hypnotherapy*; in hypnotherapy the patient is usually taken into a state of deep relaxation through guided imagery. In some cases, the patients choose their own images; others want the hypnotherapist to choose the images and take over the process.

Theodore Barber, an American hypnotherapist, has researched the use of hypnosis in treating tension headaches. Barber induces a deep relaxation state in his patients, then he goes over the conditions they have discussed such as a quarrel with a family member, deadlines at work, a traffic jam, that preceded the headache. The therapist suggests that next time one of these situations occurs, the patient will relax in this same way and avoid the tension that led to the headache.

Hypnotherapy is becoming more widespread but there are still fears concerning it. There is the fear of being unconscious and not remembering what has transpired in a session, divulging information that one does not want to share, and not being able to return to a "normal" state of consciousness after a session. In fact, hypnosis is simply a deep state of consciousness where the attention is highly focused much like meditation and visualization; because science has not been able to fully explain it, it still has the aura of mystery or mystique.

AUTOGENICS

Autogenics was developed by the German neurologist Johann Schultz in the 1920s. Having worked with hypnosis, Schultz noticed that people in a hypnotic trance experienced certain physical sensations—a feeling of heaviness in the limbs and torso as well as a feeling of warmth in the limbs. He designed certain exercises to induce conditions where the individual would be in a passive state, not exercising conscious will. After these preliminary exercises have been mastered, specific exercises were taught to deal with certain organic diseases such as asthma, injuries, and other conditions.

The six preliminary exercises, done in a sequence, included imagining the right arm to be heavy, feeling warmth in the arms and legs, sensing the heartbeat as calm and regular, slowing down the breathing, warming the solar plexus, and cooling the forehead. These exercises were done in sequence; often the words were shortened to give only the essence of the exercise, as "warm and heavy."

After Schultz published his work in 1932, (the first American edition was in 1959) many European and American psychotherapists and physicians tested his approach on various afflictions. Autogenic therapy helped stimulate the development of biofeedback training as well as some imagery-based therapies.

Autogenics has been successful in causing physical changes in blood pressure, blood sugar, heart rate, hormone secretion, brain waves, and white blood cell count.

After achieving physical relaxation, the individual can advance to the more subtle psychological aspects of autogenic training through which higher states of consciousness may be developed as well as a marked degree of autonomic control. Feats similar to that of Eastern yogis have been reported, such as self-anesthetization against a third-degree burn produced by a lighted cigarette on the back of a hand. The appeal of autogenic training to many Westerners is that it begins on an easily understandable level and slowly progresses to a more esoteric one.

BIOFEEDBACK

Biofeedback developed as a result of investigating various emotional states and feelings that affect heart rate, blood pressure, brain waves, muscle tension, and skin temperature. These conditions have been classified as "involuntary" and considered beyond the control of an individual. However, with the use of computers, auditory and visual information about these biological states could be provided to human subjects. With self-monitoring through the use of these machines, subjects could exert control over their own physiology.

Devices are used to detect heart rate, EEG alpha waves, skin resistance, finger temperature, and blood pressure. An example of this in regard to blood pressure is a blood pressure cuff wrapped around the upper arm while a microphone is placed over the artery. The cuff is inflated to the point at which a sound is picked up from the microphone, which is then amplified and fed back to the patient's earphones. The patient hears tones whenever blood pressure is just above the cuff pressure level. Instructions are provided on how to reduce the frequency of tones. When the electronic circuitry detects a sound, it automatically reduces the cuff pressure; when it hasn't detected a sound for a few seconds, it increases the cuff pressure slightly. This process keeps the cuff pressure oscillating to a point at which half of the heartbeats are heard and half are too low to be detected. To the degree that the patient is able to lower the point of oscillation, she has lowered her own blood pressure.

Among those who pioneered biofeedback techniques were Elmer and Alyce Green, who wrote the book, *Beyond Biofeedback*. Biofeedback techniques were also pioneered by Dr. Joe Kamiya in San Francisco. He monitored a subject's alpha rhythms (the waves that are generated in physical relaxation when the mind empties) with an EEG (electroencephalogram) device. When alpha rhythms were being generated, a pleasant sound would be produced.

Alpha waves are related to a feeling of well-being and most subjects were able to reach that state.

In addition to the EEG to measure brain waves, biofeedback also uses the ESR (electrical skin resistance meter), which indicates physical arousal and relaxation. This is connected to the palm of the hand, and the meter readings relate to the behavior of the autonomic system. The rate of blood flow varies with body tone and causes a change of polarization of the sweat gland membranes. The polarization varies according to how tense or relaxed one is. Stress increases the blood pressure, heart rate, the amount of muscle tension, and oxygen usage. Relaxation increases circulation to skin and organs, and lowers heart rate and muscle tension.

Biofeedback has been used successfully in treating hypertension, migraines and tension headaches, cardiac arrhythmias, and epilepsy. A friend of mine used biofeedback equipment to learn to control his respiration rate and was able to get rid of his asthma attacks. Whenever he felt an attack coming on, he would place himself in a state of meditation and monitor his respiration rate; then he was able to slow it down.

For people who like scientific proof, biofeedback equipment demonstrates how effective techniques such as relaxation, meditation, and visualization are in changing our physiological responses.

TRANSPERSONAL PSYCHOLOGY AND SOMATIC THERAPY

Transpersonal psychology includes psychological therapies whose purpose is beyond alleviating suffering and overcoming psychological disabilities. Transpersonal therapies focus on the part of us that is more than just the ego, I, or personal self; its goal is to connect us to a spiritual reality and to remove any blocks that we might have in accessing it.

The techniques employed in transpersonal psychology are different from purely mental psychotherapies. The methods are both more primal and more spiritual. *Holotropic breathwork*, developed by Stan and Christina Grof, incorporates ancient yogic breathing techniques; visualization and imagery invite the client to experience the right brain instead of simply analyzing dreams through the left brain techniques in psychoanalysis. Psychotherapists practicing the transpersonal approach recommend meditation, visualization, working with dreams, imagery, and other related techniques. Clients often attain a sense of well-being through transpersonal therapies, with new insights and spiritual and philosophical approaches to life, as well as psychic wholeness.

Many individual healers have combined physical therapies with a transpersonal psychological approach. These practices have been referred to as *Somatics* or *Somatic therapy*. Thomas Hanna (author of *The Body of Life*, *The End of Tyranny*, and *Bodies in Revolt—A Primer in Somatic Therapy*) was the first in the United States to use the term Somatics; Hanna studied with Moshe Feldenkrais and utilized Feldenkrais' practices, adding his own insights and exercises. I personally had some sessions with Tom Hanna before his tragic automobile accident in July 1990. He always emphasized new ways of thinking by the way he moved the body in different ways. Stanley Keleman, a Berkeley therapist, practiced somatic therapies and wrote many books including: *Sexuality, Self, and Survival* (1975), and *Somatic Reality: Bodily Experience and Emotional Truth* (1979).

One of the key concepts of somatics therapy is that stressors that are unexpressed are stored as muscular tensions and chemical changes in the body. By releasing the tensions, and by using techniques to reverse the chemical changes such as relaxation, the body releases the original emotions stored at the time of the trauma. Somatic disciplines seek to cultivate sensory and kinesthetic awareness, control of autonomic processes, coordination of particular muscle groups, new patterns of movement, handling of stress, and control of emotions and mental processes. Some of the better known somatic practices include the Alexander technique, Feldenkrais work, Reichian therapy, and Dreambody therapy. The Alexander technique and Feldenkrais work are a combination of bodywork and exercises; their focus is to break up old patterns in the brain by placing the body in new postures. Shamanic techniques, which have been part of traditional cultures for thousands of years, incorporate somatic disciplines.

The Alexander Technique

Frederick Matthias Alexander was an Australian actor who cured himself from voice loss when doctors were unable to help him. He observed his muscular tensions, often with mirrors, and found that the way he pulled his head backwards and downwards created his voice loss. Alexander developed educational methods to promote kinesthetic awareness and to change postural patterns that prevent optimal functioning. His approach begins by focusing attention on the relations between head and torso; his series of exercises ultimately involve the whole body.

Working with the Alexander technique has provided many health benefits in relieving pressure on certain organs such as the lungs or digestive organs as well as certain muscle systems. It also catalyzes individuals to break old patterns of thinking and emotional responses by changing their body structure. Consequently, the individual attains more freedom and ease, as well as self-confidence, from the organic flowing movements.

Alexander influenced many individuals including Moshe Feldenkrais, Wilhelm Reich, Aldous Huxley, and other well-known psychotherapists and philosophers.

The Feldenkrais Method

Moshe Feldenkrais, like Alexander, was influenced in developing his somatic discipline by his own disability—a knee injury. Through studies of anatomy, physiology, and psychology, Feldenkrais rehabilitated himself without surgery, and developed his own educational method.

The Feldenkrais Method uses movement as the starting point for releasing stored stress; through initiating new motor patterns (new habits of movement), one can break down old patterns of thinking and emotional relating. The first part of Feldenkrais' work includes hands-on bodywork known as *functional integration*. The practitioner helps the client become aware of old patterns of movement by introducing new ways of moving and experiencing the body. *Awareness Through Movement* is the second part of Feldenkrais' work; this includes exercises in which different parts of the body are moved in new ways. Each exercise is performed very slowly so that the student may experience the difference in sensation and alignment.

Individuals have gained more flexibility, vitality, relaxation, and self-awareness by working with the Feldenkrais Method. Serious structural problems have been alleviated over time by reprogramming the mind, along with the body.

Reichian Therapy

Wilhelm Reich was an Austrian-born disciple of Sigmund Freud who believed that the body's energy, which he called *orgone*, could be trapped in muscular contractions, which he referred to as the *armor* of the body. Reich's aim in breaking chronic muscular armoring was to permit the release of repressed emotions and to re-establish the free flow of orgone.

Reich believed that a patient was not fully cured until she or he achieved deep gratification in sexual intercourse. He felt that all individuals could experience an *orgasm reflex*, a spontaneous pulsation of the entire body at the time of orgasm, allowing a full energetic discharge. According to Reich, rigidities in the personality, which he referred to as *character armor*, prevent the potential for full orgasm. He worked with changing posture, gestures, and facial expressions, which maintain the personality structure.

There are many Reichian-based therapies today; the two most commonly practiced are *orgonomy* and *bioenergetics.*

An *orgonomy* session consists of a patient lying on a couch (usually in a thin gown) discussing the present issues in her/his life. The patient is encouraged to do some deep breathing and afterwards there could be some work on the body armor from the head to pelvis, combined with emotional release and discussion.

Bioenergetics was developed by Alexander Lowen, a pupil of Reich. Lowen used breathing techniques, body postures, and exercises to help people become aware of their patterns of tension. Bioenergetics deals with the relationship between somatic functions and psychological trauma. It seeks to bring about a healthy integration of body and mind so that energy is freed for pleasure rather than used in a defensive manner. The techniques utilized work on releasing physical tensions while dealing with psychological problems.

Three areas included in bioenergetics work are grounding, breathing, and character structure. *Grounding* is related to emotional security and personal authority. To be in a particular stance with feet firmly on the ground allows the energy to flow. When one has insecurity problems or problems with authority, there will be difficulty grounding.

Breathing patterns are unconsciously established over the years and caused by chronic muscle tension, often due to emotional suffering. Developing loose and flowing breathing charges the body with energy and releases many old patterns.

Character structure is the third aspect of bioenergetics, which divides the personality into five different types and relates certain emotional patterns to muscular tendencies in the way the body is held. Through getting in touch with these emotions and changing them, a new way of body posturing evolves.

Dreambody Therapy

Dreambody therapy is a *process-oriented psychology* (a process-oriented psychology is one that uses experiential techniques, emotionally and physically) that works with the relationship between dreams and problems with the physical body. All of our body features and symptoms are mirrored in our dreams; if we take the time to study our dreams and work with the symbols, there is much we can learn about the causes behind our symptoms. The symbols may not necessarily appear in our dreams but may occur in a poem, as a movement we tend to do, as voices that speak to us. Usually these symbols represent locked up feelings that have become somatized.

Arnold Mindell has developed Dreambody therapy as a tool for working with physical symptoms. He has written about it in several books, including

Working with the Dreaming Body. After discussing the symbols with his patients, Mindell has them amplify their physical symptoms. For example, a patient with stomach cramps would exaggerate them and let them become very intense in order to understand what feelings were locked up in the body. Then, after understanding the source of the blockage, the symptoms usually become more manageable and could, over time, disappear.

Dreambody therapy involves a lot of acting out with the patient and the therapist, often with the therapist taking the role of the restrictive force that has kept the emotion blocked and, consequently, the physical condition present. It is one of the most effective process-oriented therapies.

PAST LIFE THERAPY AND REGRESSION

A step beyond process-oriented psychology is *past life therapy.* Often there is trauma and anxiety still remaining in our ethereal body from experiences in other life times. (The ethereal body affects the cellular structure and function of the physical body.) If we can re-experience the events, however painful, we can often let go of the energy in our bodies, which may be tied up as a particular symptom or disease process.

Past life regression is not a form of therapy to which everyone is receptive. Some individuals are able to be regressed easier than others because they have practiced meditation and visualization techniques. The client is placed in a deep meditative state through the use of relaxation and guided imagery techniques. The therapist or facilitator may guide the client to another time or place where she is familiar with the terrain, people, or situation. From these events, the client senses the role she played and becomes emotionally involved. Often painful or joyous feelings emerge from the experience. When the client is brought back to the waking state, she often understands what her role was in that lifetime and what relationship it has to this present life.

After having several past life regressions, an emotional pattern often emerges for the client. This may be considered a root pattern, which the individual is working on over a series of lifetimes. Understanding this root emotional pattern can be extremely helpful in releasing blocks in the cellular body which are connected to physical symptoms.

I myself have conducted many past life regressions for clients, including those with chronic physical symptoms. Many changes have occurred for the individuals after only one or two sessions. One of the strongest experiences for me has been in working with women who have had difficulty conceiving. Through understanding some of the traumas they experienced as mothers or in childbirth itself, many fears were released which then enabled them to conceive and sustain a healthy pregnancy.

SHAMANIC TECHNIQUES

Shamanism is related to the Western occult tradition through alchemy. The Alchemists were interested in transformation and cultivated this through dreams, visions, and guided imagery—as well as through transmutation of plants, minerals, and other substances. Alchemists often prescribed remedies and worked with individuals by connecting to their dreams and visions.

Although *shamanic techniques* are different from alchemy, shamanism aims at alleviating physical problems through journeying and soul retrieval. In the shamanic tradition, the source of the illness is not something external which needs to be eradicated as a germ or bacteria that has entered the body. Shamans believe malefic conditions of the spirit manifest in destructive bodily and psychological conditions. These conditions are caused by individuals having lost their original spirit and allowing intrusions into the body, whether it is a disease or an evil spirit. To this end, shamans assist individuals in journeying to find their power animal or totem, and they journey themselves to help bring back parts of the soul that have been lost (*soul retrieval*). They may also use physical techniques as having patients drink some herbs that will make them "throw up" their disease, be it a germ or an entity. In addition, some shamans employ a sucking technique where they suck out the disease and then spit it up. It is essential, of course, that the patients believe in the shaman's healing powers and agree to become empowered and free of disease.

CHAPTER 5:
TRADITIONAL
CHINESE MEDICINE

Traditional Chinese Medicine (TCM) is a very broad system that includes work with the energy body and *chi* as well as the spiritual, psychological, and emotional causes of disease. Chinese Herbology also deals with the physical body, helping to cleanse toxic organs and re-balance various systems.

TCM is based on the belief that all humanity is a part of the natural environment and that health or balance can only be achieved when one follows natural law, adapting to the changes of the seasons and the surrounding environment. Chinese medicine has its philosophical basis in *Taoism* (the Way of the Tao, or the Way of Life). Taoism teaches that all phenomena exist within interrelated space. It also expounds that everything has an energy field or vibration and is in a constant state of flux.

What activates all phenomena is the movement of energy between two poles, *yin* and *yang*. Yin is the tendency toward contraction and centripetality; yang, the tendency towards expansion and centrifugality. Yin is receptive and feminine; yang, active and masculine. Yin is the Earth force; yang is the force of Heaven. The Chinese character for yin refers to the shady side of a slope. It is associated with qualities like cold, rest, passivity, darkness, interiority, downwardness, inwardness, and decrease. The character for yang is the sunny side of a slope. It is associated with heat, stimulation, movement, activity, excitement, vigor, light, upwardness, outwardness, and increase.

The front part of the body is considered yin and the back, yang. The upper part is more yang than the lower part. Illnesses that are characterized by weakness, slowness, coldness, and underactivity are yin. Illnesses that manifest strength, forceful movements, heat, and overactivity are yang.

This chapter discusses some of the most important concepts in Chinese medicine, and provides information on diagnosis and treatment.

CHI

The dynamic vital energy present in all things is called *chi* by the Chinese. When a person is in good health or balance (physically, emotionally, and spiritually), her chi is maximized, and she resonates with the environment. When out of balance, her chi is low or deficient.

The Chinese have three sources of chi. Original or *pre-natal chi* is transmitted by parents to children; this is the inherited constitution. The second source is *grain chi*, derived from the digestion of food. The third is the *natural air chi*, which is extracted by the lungs from the air we breathe.

Chi has five major functions in the body. The first is movement (including involuntary movements and activities like thinking and dreaming). Chi is in constant motion in the body. Secondly, chi protects the body from pathological and environmental agents. Thirdly, chi transforms food into blood and urine. It also governs retention of the body's substance by holding organs in their proper place and preventing excessive loss of bodily fluids. Finally, chi warms the body.

BLOOD

Blood in Chinese medicine is a broader concept than in Western medicine. Its main activity is to circulate throughout the body, nourishing and maintaining its various parts. Blood moves through the blood vessels and also the meridians. It originates through the transformation of food. After the stomach receives food, the spleen distills a purified essence from it. The spleen transports this essence up to the lungs. Here it is combined with air to form blood, which is then propelled through the body by the heart chi in combination with the chest chi.

The heart, liver, and spleen all have special relationships to the blood. Blood depends on the heart for its continuous circulation throughout the body. The liver stores the inactive blood, and the spleen keeps it within the blood vessels.

JING

Jing or "essence" is the substance that underlies all organic life. Jing is like a fluid and is the basis of reproduction and development. Pre-natal jing is the essence we inherit from our parents, and post-natal jing is derived from the purified parts of ingested food.

Jing is the material that imbues an organism with development from conception to birth. Disharmonies of jing might involve improper motivation, sexual dysfunction, and premature aging. Jing is different from chi in that chi is involved with movement, but jing is associated with the slow movement of organic change.

SHEN

Shen means "spirit"; it is the substance of human life. Shen is associated with the ability to think, to discriminate, and to choose. Shen also has a material aspect. It is the mind's ability to form ideas and the desire of the personality to live. When shen is out of harmony, one's thinking may be muddled or one may suffer from insomnia, unconsciousness, or incoherent speech.

ORGANS

The Chinese organs are different from the Western organs in that they are defined by their *function*, not their structure. The Chinese recognize the *triple burner* as an organ, but it is not a physical entity. The triple burner is a relationship between various organs that regulate water. It is the pathway that makes these organs a complete system; since fire controls water, the triple burner implies fire.

Organs are divided into yin and yang. The function of the yin organs is to produce, transform, regulate, and store the fundamental substances—chi, blood, jing, shen, and fluids. The function of the yang organs is to receive, break down, and absorb that part of the food that will be transformed into fundamental substance and excrete the unused part.

Yin Organs	Yang Organs
heart	small intestine
lungs	large intestine
spleen	stomach
liver	gall bladder
kidneys	bladder
pericardium	triple burner

MERIDIANS AND ACUPUNCTURE

Meridians are the channels that carry chi and blood through the body; they connect the interior of the body with the exterior. The philosophy of acupuncture is that working with points on the outside of the body affects the substances that are traveling through the meridians.

The meridian system is comprised of the twelve regular meridians that correspond to the six yin and six yang organs. There are also eight extra meridians, only two of which, the *Governing vessel* and the *Conception vessel*, are considered major meridians. They have points that are not on any of the twelve regular meridians. The paths of the other six meridians intersect with the twelve meridians and have no independent points.

Disorder within a meridian creates disharmony on its pathway and could result in problems in the meridian's connecting organ. For example, disorder in the stomach meridian may cause a toothache in the upper gums because the meridian passes through this area. Disharmony in an organ may also manifest in the corresponding meridian. Understanding the connections between the substances, organs, and meridians is the essence of Chinese medicine. Chinese medicine uses acupuncture and herbs to re-balance yin and yang in the meridians and organs. An example of imbalance is excess anger, which would indicate too much liver chi.

The idea behind acupuncture is that the insertion of fine needles into points along the meridians can re-balance bodily disharmonies. The action of the needle affects the chi and the blood in the meridians, thus affecting the substances and organs. The needles help to reduce excesses, increase deficiencies, warm cold areas, cool down hot areas, circulate stagnant energy, and move congealed energy. There are about 365 points on the surface meridians of the body, but in practice, a doctor may use only about 150 points. Each acupuncture point has a defined therapeutic action—a combination of points is, therefore, always chosen. Needles are made of stainless steel and produce relatively little pain when inserted. The depth to which a needle penetrates depends on the particular point.

In addition to acupuncture, a related technique called *moxibustion* is employed. Moxibustion applies the heat from burning substances at certain acupuncture points. The heating substance, or *moxa*, is mugwort (artemisia vulgaris). This helps to increase the effect of the acupuncture treatment.

HERBOLOGY

Chinese Herbology is an extensive body of knowledge that has been developed over several millennia into an organized system of medicine. Substances used in the Chinese materia medica span a great range of materials, from herbs and minerals to strange animal products. Each entry is usually defined in terms of how the various herbs and their combinations affect imbalances in the body.

There are many classical prescriptions that can re-balance disharmonies in the body. These prescriptions are found in the pharmacopoeias and manuals. Most of the herbs are used as teas, but herbal tablets, powders, and tinctures are also utilized.

PATTERNS OF DISEASE

The Chinese do not speak of causes of disease in the same way as does Western medicine. Cause implies a linear progression; Chinese medicine works in a "circular" way, believing that there are many factors that create a pattern of imbalance, disharmony, or dis-ease. These factors are categorized under environment, emotional outlook, and way of life.

Environmental factors are spoken of as the "six pernicious influences." These six are Wind, Cold, Fire or Heat, Dryness, Dampness, and Summer Heat. When weakened by an imbalance of yin and yang, a climatic phenomenon can invade the body. If the protective chi is strong, the influence is expelled and the individual recovers. But if the chi is weak, the influence may go deep and become involved with the internal organs. Illnesses generated by any of the "pernicious factors" can come on suddenly. When the pernicious influences arise internally, symptoms come on gradually. This is the case with chronic disease as opposed to acute disease.

All the climatic influences are images for body processes. The body does not have to experience damp climate to have damp in the lungs; our emotional and mental states can create the same condition.

SEVEN EMOTIONS

The seven emotions that particularly affect the body are joy, anger, sadness, grief, pensiveness (worry), fear, and fright. Sadness and grief as well as fear and fright are often combined as one emotion. The seven emotions correspond to the five yin organs:

heart—joy
liver—anger
lungs—sadness and grief
spleen—pensiveness or worry
kidneys—fear and fright

The two organs most susceptible to emotions are the heart and the liver. The heart stores the shen; imbalances may lead to insomnia, crying or laughing, and extreme hysteria. Imbalances in the liver can result in excess anger or emotional frustration.

Organ	Out of Balance	In Balance
liver, gall bladder	anger	patience
heart, small intestine	excitement	joy
spleen, stomach	worry	sympathy
kidney, bladder	fear	confidence
lung, large intestine	grief	happiness

WAY OF LIFE

Several factors that the Chinese refer to as *Way of Life* are important in determining a person's state of health. These include diet, sexual activity, and physical activity. Diet is important because the stomach receives food and the spleen transforms it into chi and blood. Preference for certain types of food can cause disharmonies. For example, too much raw food can strain the yang aspect of the spleen and generate intense cold. Fatty and greasy foods can produce dampness and heat.

Many of the principles of Chinese medicine have been utilized by the Japanese philosopher George Ohsawa in creating the Macrobiotic Diet. Macrobiotics, however, is not a part of Chinese medicine though it is often practiced and used along with acupuncture and herbs (see Chapter 9).

Excessive sexual activity is often considered a precipitating factor of disease. Overindulgence affects the kidneys and reduces vitality; giving birth too many times weakens the jing and the blood.

Physical activity is important, but excess can strain the spleen's ability to produce chi and blood. Inactivity can weaken the vitality of chi and blood; excess use of a part of the body can also weaken it.

THE FOUR EXAMINATIONS

Before making a diagnosis, the Chinese physician performs four examinations—Looking, Listening and Smelling, Asking, and Touching.

In the Looking examination, the first factor is the patient's general appearance: how she looks, her manner and the state of her shen. Lack of interest, apathy, and depression can indicate an imbalanced shen. The second factor is facial color. The third concerns the tongue, including the material of the tongue itself, its coating, and its shape and movement. The fourth is the bodily secretions and excretions.

A person whose appearance is strong is more likely to have disharmonies of excess. One who is frail and weak-looking will tend to have disharmonies of deficiency. One who is agitated, talkative, aggressive, and unstable usually manifests a yang tendency. A more inward, quiet manner is usually yin. The color of the face and its moistness are related to the chi and blood. If the face is healthy, the indications are that the chi and the blood are not weakened and the illness is not serious.

Tongue observation is a central point of the Four Examinations. The tongue can be various shades of red and can have varying degrees of moisture. A normal tongue is pale red and somewhat moist, which indicates that the chi and blood are normal. A pale tongue indicates deficient blood or chi or excess cold. A red tongue points to a heat condition in the body.

The coating on the surface of the tongue is the result of spleen activity. During its vaporization of essences, the spleen causes small amounts of impure substances to ascend which come out on the tongue. This is related to digestion. The coating varies in thickness, color, and appearance.

The most important of the examinations is touching, and it consists of pulse taking. Chinese medicine takes the pulses at the radial artery near the wrist. Many years of experience are required to get the feel of the differences between pulses. The three middle fingers are used, one at each position near the radial artery. The pulse is palpitated at three levels of pressure—first, a light superficial touch, then a moderate amount of pressure is applied, and third, a very deep pressure. A balanced pulse is felt mostly at the middle level. Normal speed is between 4 and 5 beats per complete respiration (one inhale and one exhale), which amounts to 70–75 beats per minute. A normal pulse may vary according to the type of work a person does, her age, and body type such as thin or heavy. Chinese texts describe about twenty-eight different types of pulses, though most people are a combination of types.

THE FIVE PHASES

The five phases in Chinese philosophy and medicine have been misunderstood in the Western world. They are commonly referred to as the Five Elements, which is an incorrect translation; they are five *movements* or phases. The phases are a system of correspondences that explain the dynamics of events or relationships. Each phase describes certain functions and qualities. The phase called *Wood* is associated with active functions that are in a growing phase. *Fire* designates functions that have reached a maximal state of activity and are about to begin a decline or resting period. *Earth* designates balance or neutrality. *Metal* represents functions in a declining state. *Water* represents functions that have reached a normal state of rest and are about to change the direction of their activity.

The five phases were originally related to the seasons with Wood-Spring, Fire-Summer, Earth-Indian summer, Metal-Autumn, and Water-Winter. In time, they were related to color, odor, emotions; and many other correspondences were added. They were also associated with the organs, and thus they became connected with the system of Chinese medicine.

The organs are placed in the five phases in what is known as the *Mutual Control* or *Mutual Checking* sequence. In this sequence, each organ controls the next one so that there will not be any excesses or deficiencies. Thus, Wood-liver controls Earth-spleen, which controls Water-kidneys, which controls Fire-heart, which controls Metal-lungs. Disharmonies may be produced if Wood does not produce enough Fire, which means the liver is not sending blood to the heart, or if Wood overcontrols the spleen, which indicates excess blood from the liver invading the spleen.

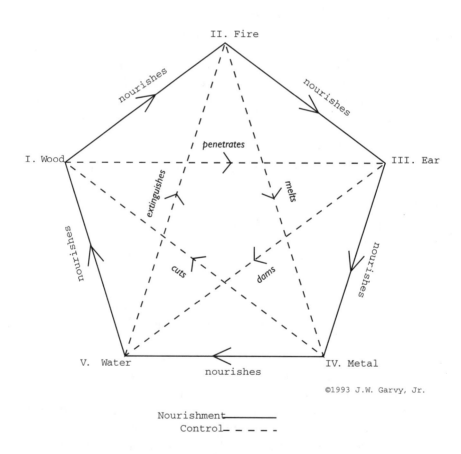

©1993 J.W. Garvy, Jr.

Nourishment ———————
Control _ _ _ _ _

Cycles of Nourishment & Control

FIVE PHASE CORRESPONDENCES

	I. WOOD	II. FIRE	III. EARTH	IV. METAL	V. WATER
Function	Purification	Circulation	Digestion	Respiration	Elimination
Organ/Solid	Liver	Heart	Spleen/Pancreas	Lungs	Kidneys
Organ/Hollow	Gallbladder	Small	Stomach	Large Intestine	Bladder
Color	Green	Red	Yellow (Orange)	White	Gray, Deep Blue, Brown, Black
Flavor	Sour	Bitter	Sweet	Hot, Pungent	Salty
Emotion	Anger	Joy	Sympathy	Grief	Fear
Sound	Shouting	Laughter	Singing	Weeping	Groaning
Direction	Up	Outward	Horizontal	Down	Inward
Sense	Sight	Touch/Speech	Taste	Smell	Hearing
Head Part	Eyes	Tongue	Mouth	Nose	Ears
Secretion	Tears	Sweat	Saliva	Nasal Fluid	Urine
Season	Spring	Summer	Indian Summer	Autumn	Winter
Climate	Wind	Heat	Dampness	Dryness	Cold
Injuries	Back of Neck	Mouth	Feet	Nose	Shins

CHAPTER 6:
AYURVEDIC MEDICINE

Like Traditional Chinese Medicine, the system of Ayurvedic medicine, the ancient Hindu healing system, has been in existence for thousands of years. Its techniques also work with all of Paracelsus' causes of disease, from disturbance of the magnetic field to spiritual and emotional causes, to physical toxins, and imbalance.

Ayurvedic medicine views health as a continuous relationship between the individual and the cosmos. In Sanskrit, *ayas* means "life" or "daily living"; *veda* means "knowledge." The science of Ayurveda encompasses many diagnostic techniques (pulse diagnosis, nail diagnosis, facial diagnosis); various types of cleansing; herbs and homeopathic remedies; an extensive dietary regimen based on the different tastes and their attributes; as well as yoga postures, various *mudras* (hand gestures) and *mantras* (chants) that help balance out specific energies. It is a comprehensive and holistic system.

The *theory of the five elements* forms the basis for the Ayurvedic system. *Ether* is the first element; it is the medium through which sound is transmitted and is related to the ear and the actions of speech and hearing. *Air* is created from Ether and refers to the sense of touch and the skin. The organ for the sense of touch is the hand and its action is holding. *Fire* or heat came about through the friction of Ether. Fire manifests as light, heat, and color and is related to vision. (The eye—the organ of sight—governs the action of walking.) Through the heat of Fire, certain elements dissolved and liquefied (*Water*), and solidified to form *Earth*. Water is related to taste and the tongue. The tongue in Ayurvedic medicine is associated with the genitals—the clitoris and penis, and the action of procreation. Earth refers to the sense of smell, and the nose—the sensory organ of smell—is associated with the anus and the action of excretion.

TRIDOSHA

Ayurvedic medicine is organized around three humors or *doshas* which form the core of the system.

Vata is the first dosha; it is the principle of movement and is formed from Ether and Air. Vata governs breathing, movements of the muscles and tissues, pulsations in the heart, expansion and contraction, as well as the motion of cytoplasm and impulses to nerve cells. Feelings and emotions governed by Vata include nervousness, fear, anxiety, pain, tremors, and spasms. The large intestine, pelvic cavity, bones, skin, ears, and thighs are the seats of Vata; excesses of Vata will accumulate in these areas.

Pitta, the second humor, is formed from Fire and Water; it is akin to bile. Pitta refers to metabolism, nutrition, digestion, absorption, assimilation, body temperature, and skin coloration. Psychologically, an excess of Pitta arouses anger, hate, and jealousy. The small intestine, stomach, sweat glands, blood, fat, eyes, and skin are the seats of Pitta.

Kapha originates from Water and Earth. Kapha cements the elements in the body; it lubricates the joints, provides moisture to the skin, helps to heal wounds, and maintains immunity. Kapha is the mucus secretion present in the chest, throat, head, sinuses, nose, mouth, and joints. Psychologically, Kapha is related to the emotions of attachment, greed, and envy; it is also expressed in tendencies toward calmness, forgiveness, and love.

The *tridosha* governs all metabolic processes—anabolism or building up (Kapha), catabolism or breaking down (Vata), and metabolism (Pitta). When one dosha is out of balance, the metabolism will be disturbed.

CONSTITUTIONAL TYPES

Vata types may be too tall or too short; their complexion is dark and their skin is usually cold, dry, rough, and cracked. Hair is often curly with thin eyelashes; nails are rough and brittle and noses may be turned up. Physiological tendencies of Vata people vary. They often crave sweet, sour, and salty tastes and like hot drinks. Their urine is more scanty, and feces tend to be dry, hard, and small. They perspire less than other types. Their hands and feet are often cold, and they tend toward constipation. Vata types are alert, active, restless, sleep less, and talk fast. Their appetites are irregular; they have bursts of energy and often have difficulty sleeping. Psychologically, they have short memories but quick mental understanding. They can be nervous, fearful, and anxious at times.

Pitta types tend toward medium height. Their complexion may be yellowish or reddish with skin that is soft, warm, and less wrinkled than Vata skin. They blush easily and are sensitive to the sun. Physiologically, they have a strong metabolism and good digestion. They often crave sweet, bitter, and astringent flavors, and enjoy cold drinks. Their sleep is generally uninter-rupted. They produce a large volume of urine and their feces are liquid and soft. There may be a tendency toward excessive perspiring. Body temperature runs high and hands and feet tend to be warm. Psychologically, they have good powers of comprehension and are intelligent and sharp. Their emotional traits tend toward hate, anger, and jealousy. Pitta people are ambitious, like to be leaders, and display impatience.

Those of *Kapha constitution* have well-developed bodies though they tend to carry excess weight. When exercising properly, they are good athletes. Kapha types have fair and bright complexions; their skin is soft and oily and tends to be pale; their hair is thick, soft, and wavy. Physiologically, Kapha peo-ple have regular appetites—their digestion functions slowly and there is less intake of food. They tend to move slowly and crave pungent, bitter, and astrin-gent foods. Stools are soft and may be pale in color with slow evacuation. Their sleep is sound, and they possess a strong vitality with good stamina. Psychologically, Kapha types are tolerant, calm, forgiving, and loving when balanced. They may also be greedy, envious, possessive, stubborn, reactionary, and complacent. Their comprehension is slow, but they retain knowledge well. They need motivation and stimulation, just as Vatas require balance and relax-ation, and Pittas need a challenge.

Vata-Pitta people have poor circulation, characteristic of Vata types, but cannot handle heat as well due to their Pitta qualities. They often have wavy hair, resulting from Vata's curliness and Pitta's straightness. When their energy is out of balance, fear alternates with anger as a response to stress; they can be bullying and domineering. Both Vata and Pitta have lightness and intensity. When unbalanced, Vata's tendency to addiction for pain control and Pitta's intensity combine to stronger addictive states. If directed, they can work with intensive self-development. They need to be weighted down with the heavi-ness of Kapha.

Pitta-Kapha types have the stability of Kapha with the adaptability of Pitta. They usually enjoy good physical health due to Kapha's strong body, and Pitta's good metabolism. Pitta's danger can be balanced by Kapha's cautious-ness. The negative side is seen in Pitta's arrogance and Kapha's self-satisfac-tion. Both of these types have a share of oiliness or wetness and need the dryness of introspection or spiritual disciplines.

Vata-Kapha types suffer from cold; their lack of heat may manifest in digestive disorders like constipation or respiratory disease with a lot of mucus. They can be overzealous about what they do and often overdo things. Emotional hurts go deep with the strong emotional nature of Kapha and the overactive and sporadic nature of Vata.

DISEASE CLASSIFICATION

In Ayurvedic medicine, disease is classified according to its origin—psychological, spiritual, or physical. Disease is also classified according to the site of manifestation and the imbalance of the doshas—Vata, Pitta, or Kapha. Vata disease originates in the large intestine; Vata types often have gas, low back pain, arthritis, sciatica, and neuralgia. Pitta disease originates in the small intestine; these types often have gall bladder and liver disorders, ulcers, acidic conditions, and gastritis. Kapha diseases start in the stomach; they may experience tonsillitis, sinusitis, bronchitis, and congestion of the lungs.

In terms of emotions, repressed fear creates an imbalance of Vata, anger causes excess Pitta, while envy and greed aggravate Kapha. If physical conditions, improper diet, and environmental toxins create an imbalance in the body, then the corresponding emotions will also be present—distorted Vata creates fear, depression, and nervousness; excess Pitta causes anger, hate, and jealousy; and too much Kapha may create possessiveness, greed, and attachment. Fear and anxiety alter the flora of the large intestine, and problems with gas or bloating may result. Repressed anger changes the flora of the gallbladder and bile duct and may cause inflammation on the walls of the small intestine. Excess envy and greed may affect the mucous membranes of the stomach. Repressed emotions affect *agni*, the biological fire that governs metabolism. When agni is low, the body's auto-immune response is affected, and this may lead to allergies—pollens, dust, and other substances.

TREATMENT

The most important treatment in Ayurvedic medicine is the elimination of toxins through various cleansing procedures. Ayurveda uses the term *panchakarma* to include the five basic cleansing processes: vomiting, laxatives, medicated enemas, nasal administration of medicine, and purification of the blood. When there is excess mucus in the chest, bile in the small intestine, or gas accumulation in the colon, elimination therapies are helpful.

When there is congestion in the lungs causing repeated attacks of bronchitis, coughs, or asthma, *therapeutic vomiting* is used. Three or four glasses of an herb tea or two glasses of salt water is administered first. Then the tongue is rubbed to induce vomiting. Therapeutic vomiting is also indicated for skin diseases, chronic sinus problems, and chronic indigestion.

When allergies, rashes, or skin inflammations develop, it is due to bile accumulation in the gallbladder, liver, or intestines. For these conditions, Ayurveda uses *purgatives* or *laxatives*. Herbs like senna, flaxseed, and psyllium seed husks as well as castor oil are used.

Enema treatments are taken for various Vata disorders such as chronic gas, constipation, hyperacidity, arthritis, rheumatism, and gout. There are several types of enemas—oil enemas in which 1/2 cup of sesame or olive oil is heated and put into the enema bag, decoction enemas in which various herbs are decocted, and nutritive enemas where a cup of warm milk or bone marrow soup are added to the enema.

Another cleansing process involves nasal administration of medication, or *nasya*. Nasal administration helps to correct the disorders of *prana* affecting the cerebral, sensory, and motor functions. It is indicated for dryness of the nose, sinus congestion, hoarseness, migraine, as well as eye and ear problems. Breathing can also be improved through nasal massage. In this technique, the inner walls of the nostril are massaged with oils, ghee, or the juice of various herbs like gotu-kola or aloe vera.

Bloodletting is used in various Pitta disorders like rashes and acne where toxins are circulated in the bloodstream. The Ayurvedic physician extracts a small amount of blood from the vein which relieves the tension created by the toxins in the blood. Bloodletting stimulates antitoxic substances in the bloodstream which help develop the auto-immune mechanism. Blood purifying herbs include burdock root tea, saffron, turmeric, and calamus root powder.

BALANCING THE BODY

In order to balance the body, three things must be in equilibrium. These are *prana*, life force—called *chi* in Chinese medicine—which brings body, mind, and spirit together on a single strand of breath and causes them to work as a single organism; *tejas*, the force of transmutation which permits body, mind, and spirit to influence one another; and *ojas*, the subtle manifestation or the glue that cements body, mind, and spirit together. Vata, Pitta, and Kapha are the gross manifestations of prana, tejas, and ojas. When physical, mental, and spiritual digestion are at their peak, Vata, Pitta, and Kapha are produced from bodily functions.

Prana is obtained from our food and the atmosphere; breathing recharges prana; nourishment and water also carry prana. While most nutrients are absorbed from the small intestine, prana is absorbed from the colon. The health of our lungs and colon determine how much prana we can absorb. When the lungs or colon are not healthy, too much Vata is generated, which can then cause disease. Vata especially affects bone. Cigarette smokers often lose more calcium from their bones due to the effect of carbon monoxide on blood chemistry.

Tejas is fire; prana inflames tejas. When the mind is clear and stable, tejas burns cleanly; when the mind is agitated by emotion, tejas is imbalanced and produces too much Pitta. Chemical toxins are transported by the blood; the ability of tejas to nurture the digestive system depends upon the blood, the liver, and spleen—which control the blood, and the brain.

Ojas is the medium through which the force of tejas is transmitted. Ojas is a substance, which unlike prana and tejas can be produced, collected, and stored. When there is good digestion of food and other sensory impressions, ojas is efficiently produced. Ojas is a living force which protects the integrity of the individual. It has a negative counterpart called *Ama*, which is a living substance in the sense that it is a collection of nutrients for alien invaders like bacteria, viruses, and cancer cells. Ojas is the foundation of physical immunity and produces the aura. The aura is the first line of defense against intrusions and a buffer against negative vibrations.

Indigestion is the main cause of disease; physical indigestion causes mental indigestion, and vice versa; the two usually exist together. If the body is purified as much as possible, then one can begin working with the mind. Vata-caused indigestion mainly affects the large intestine. Usually, constipation alternates with loose stools, and there is intestinal gas. Pitta-caused indigestion affects mainly the small intestine and usually causes loose stools. Burning sensations such as heartburn are common. Kapha-caused indigestion affects mainly the stomach; there is usually heaviness in the upper abdomen and in the limbs, with constipation.

Ayurvedic medicine works to remove the cause of the indigestion, eliminate the excess energy from the doshas, balance the doshas, rekindle the digestive fires, and then rebuild the organism.

The first treatments concern the elimination of Ama. Fasting is the most basic way to cleanse the body. Vata types should not fast on just water for more than a day or two; they may fast on vegetable juices, or for a prolonged fast, they should choose a single food like cooked vegetables. Pitta types do well fasting on vegetable or fruit juices, or raw vegetables or fruit. Kapha people may fast on water for several days or raw vegetable and fruit juices.

Medicated enemas are an important treatment in cleansing the body. Sweats in a sauna or in a wet steam bath are beneficial, depending on which doshas are out of balance.

If the patient is strong and the disease weak, the *panchakarmas* or cleansings should be used. If the patient is weak and the disease strong, the doshas should be balanced first and the patient strengthened before doing the cleansings.

After cleansing the body, there are ways to balance the doshas. If the imbalance is due to excess Vata, tea made from ginger with ground-up fennel and dill seeds is helpful. Ginger and garlic are good to rekindle digestive fire.

Light, well-cooked foods and warm liquids are soothing. Yoga stretches are good as well as regular sunbathing. To balance excess Pitta, fennel may be used. Psyllium seed husks or bitter herbs like gentian or Oregon grape root help to light the digestive fire. Raw foods and juices with coriander and sandalwood tea are good. Also, walks in the open air and sunbathing early or late in the day are helpful. If Kapha is in excess, dry ginger, black pepper, or cumin help to digest Ama. Bitter or pungent herbs like garlic or black pepper will activate the digestive fire. Small quantities of roasted food may be taken with as little liquid as possible. Vigorous exercise and extensive sunbathing to encourage sweating is good as well as wind-bathing, with the body well-wrapped, to encourage body heat.

DIET

Ayurvedic diet is based on the individual constitution. The taste of food is taken into account—whether it is sweet, sour, salty, pungent, bitter, or astringent—and also whether it is heavy or light, hot or cold, oily or dry, liquid or solid. The seasons of the year are also considered in choosing diet. During summer when the temperature is hot, people perspire readily. Since Pitta predominates in the summer, it is not good to eat spicy, pungent foods because they aggravate this dosha. In autumn when the wind is high and dry, Vata predominates. At this time one should avoid dry fruits, high protein foods, and other foods that increase Vata. Winter is the season to avoid cold drinks, cheese, yogurt, and dairy products as they increase Kapha.

There are six basic tastes in Ayurveda: sweet, sour, salty, pungent, bitter, and astringent. These tastes are derived from the five elements. Sweet contains Earth and Water elements; sour, Earth and Fire; and salty, Water and Fire. The pungent taste contains Fire and Air; bitter, Air and Ether; and astringent, Air and Earth.

(See Chapter 8 for specific foods for Vata, Pitta, and Kapha types.)

MENTAL BALANCE

Once the body is cleansed and balanced, attention should be given to mental states. Vata types tend to worry and be fearful, so they need to keep their minds occupied. Meditation as well as being engaged in projects where they utilize mental energy is helpful. Pitta types tend to anger, especially when they are impatient. Pittas need complex projects to engage their energy so they do not become too restless. Kapha types tend to be complacent and often want to consume and possess things. They also become lazy in caring for their health. It is important for them to be strongly motivated and to concentrate on one activity at a time.

YOGA

The practice of yoga works with Ayurveda in maintaining health and preventing disease. Yoga postures and exercise balance the nervous system, improve the metabolism, and help the body to handle stress. Certain postures move accumulated energies that have stagnated in various organs of the body. Ayurveda indicates which type of yoga is suitable for individuals according to their constitutions. (See Chapter 12 for more details on yoga.)

PART III:
THERAPIES TO
CLEANSE AND
BALANCE THE
PHYSICAL BODY

CHAPTER 7:
CLEANSING
AND ELIMINATION

Paracelsus stated that the fourth and fifth causes of disease are the introduction into the body of harmful substances, and wrong physical habits. Since the physical body is our vehicle for living on this earth—the temple that allows us to do our work in this lifetime—it needs to be nurtured and cleansed.

The spiral of healing moves from the etheric body to the physical and from the physical, back to the etheric and higher bodies. Our Western medical tradition, so strongly influenced by Christian philosophy, which denies and subjugates the flesh, feeds the body chemical medicines, removes parts of the body unnecessarily, and has no awareness of cleansing or natural healing practices.

Any harmful substance we eat, drink, or breathe into our bodies will either be removed by the body or else stored. Over time, this is bound to be harmful. Even if we eat only organic foods, we may eat foods that are inappropriate for our individual metabolisms; if so, the body will need re-balancing. This chapter covers cleansing and elimination—helpful remedies to use when we have introduced harmful substances into our bodies, as well as good preventive medicine—and the following chapters provide guidance on ensuring that we give our bodies the foods they need, herbal medicines that do not cause new symptoms when we are ill, and exercise.

Examining ancient traditions of healing, Ayurvedic medicine has a series of cleansing modalities known as *panchakarmas* that cleanse the intestines, the nasal passages, the skin, and other orifices used for elimination. Traditional Chinese Medicine also has many herbal formulas and other techniques for cleansing.

Since the 1960s, many ways to cleanse the body have been uncovered from ancient sources and are available to those who practice natural healing.

In order for the body to function properly and to metabolize and absorb nutrients from foods and dietary supplements, the colon must be cleansed regularly. Whereas the upper portion of the digestive system—mouth, stomach, and small intestine—is designed for absorption, the lower part—the colon or large intestine—is for elimination; it contains a number of microorganisms, known as intestinal flora, which are essential for proper elimination.

Failure to eliminate waste products from the body causes fermentation and putrefaction, leading to many health problems. When eating several meals a day, it is impossible not to have residues accumulate in the colon in the form of undigested food particles. Food waste can build up in the cells and tissues, which become toxic if they continue to ferment and putrefy. The purpose of the colon as an organ of elimination is to collect waste material from every part of the body and, through the peristaltic action of the colon's muscles, remove the waste. If it is allowed to accumulate, disease and imbalance may occur.

Constipation is a major condition underlying many health problems. A state of constipation often exists when movements of the bowel appear to be normal, but there is an accumulation of feces somewhere in the colon. Constipation involves not only the retention of feces in the bowel, but also the retention of feces in the first half of the colon (from the cecum to the middle of the transverse colon).

The wall of the first section of the colon has nerves and muscles which create wavelike motions known as *peristalsis* to move the contents of the colon from the cecum to the rectum. The first half of the colon also extracts any nutritional material which the small intestine was unable to gather. This material is collected by the blood vessels lining the walls of the colon and carried to the liver for processing. If the feces in the colon have fermented, any nutritional elements present pass into the bloodstream as polluted products (referred to as *toxemia*, a condition in which the blood contains poisonous products which are produced by the growth of pathogenic or disease-producing bacteria).

The other important function of the first half of the colon is to gather (from the glands in its walls) the intestinal flora needed to lubricate the colon. Many people believe that colon irrigations and enemas wash out the intestinal flora and deprive the colon of lubrication. Actually, this is not true. When the accumulation of feces in the bowel leads to blockage or encrustation, it is not possible for the lining of the colon to function normally, and the glands cannot produce the necessary lubrication. The encrustation interferes with the intestinal flora necessary for colon lubrication and the absorption of nutritional elements from the small intestine.

A colon irrigation or colonic is a way of bringing water to the colon so that the fecal lining is soaked and saturated in order for its removal to take place gradually. While the patient lies relaxed on a table which is connected to the colonic equipment, a colon therapist controls the water flow and also massages the colon to help loosen encrusted fecal matter. A colonic takes about forty minutes to an hour; during that time 20 or 30 gallons of water are inserted into the colon through the rectum and then expelled. Initially, most people need at least three colonics, about one or two weeks apart. These treatments should be continued every few months to permit maximum absorption of food.

In studying a diagram of the colon, each section of the colon corresponds to another organ within the body. Cleansing the colon helps in de-toxifying the other organs as well.

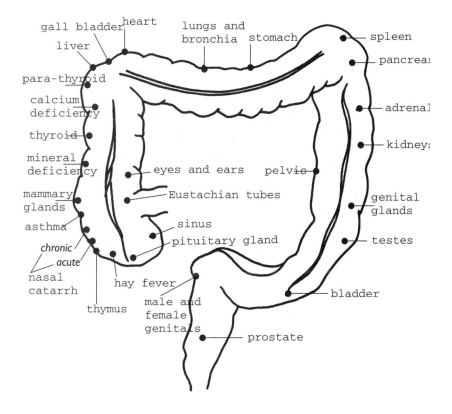

Normal Colon with Anatomical Centers

Many diseases and conditions of body imbalance are related to blockage of fecal material within the colon. One of these is diarrhea, a frequent fluid evacuation of the bowel. There are several types of diarrhea. The most common is *inflammatory* diarrhea caused by congestion of mucus in the colon; another type is *pancreatic,* due to a disturbance of the pancreas; there is also *parasitic* diarrhea which is incited by the presence of intestinal parasites. All of these are helped by colonic treatments.

Metabolic diseases are extremely common in the United States and Europe. Hypoglycemia (low blood sugar), diabetes, thyroid imbalance (conditions of being overweight and underweight are usually related to the thyroid), and the various diseases we refer to as cancer. The body's metabolism is dependent upon the hormone thyroxin for its proper function; iodine is the basic ingredient of this hormone. The ability of the thyroid to utilize iodine is commensurate with the lack of toxicity in the colon. When the thyroid is unable to generate sufficient thyroxin, hair may turn gray, skin often becomes dry or brittle, body weight increases, and there is a loss of vitality.

The *pancreas* is an organ intimately connected with the metabolism of blood sugar and the digestive process. Pancreatic juice contains digestive enzymes and is alkaline in its reaction, so it establishes the right conditions for the intestinal enzymes to function in the small intestine. Towards the middle of the pancreas there is a group of glands called the *islets of Langerhans,* which produce insulin, the hormone responsible for regulating the metabolism of sugar and other carbohydrates. When the body is toxic and there is fermentation in the colon, these glands are unable to produce the needed insulin. If not enough insulin is produced, sugar is increased in the blood and discharged into the kidneys, a condition referred to as diabetes.

Working along with the pancreas is the *liver;* it is involved with fat and protein metabolism. The liver produces bile, which is stored in the gallbladder and helps to break down fats in the body. Being the largest organ, the liver is a strong detoxifying agent and needs to be cleansed along with the colon.

One simple way of detoxifying the liver is through bitter foods and herbs. Both the Ayurvedic system and the traditional Chinese system incorporate foods and herbs with a bitter taste.

Eating dark green vegetables such as mustard greens, collard greens, turnip greens, dandelion greens, arugula, and kale at least once a day aid the liver as well as providing more minerals and vitamins than any other foods. Liquid chlorophyll is also helpful in de-toxifying the liver as well as being the carrier of the magnesium ion. An excellent herb for the liver and digestive system in general is golden seal leaf (not the root or powder); golden seal leaf is bitter and works to cleanse the liver. In Traditional Chinese Medicine one speaks of "too much liver heat." This is true of those whose liver is toxic; their symptoms may be strong allergic reactions such as skin irritations, runny nose and eyes, and wheezing. Women who experience intense hot flashes also need to cleanse their liver. I have found this particular herb to work better for these conditions than any other Western herb. Another bitter herb is Oregon grape root, which is dark yellow in color, and helps to cleanse the liver as well as produce more bile.

To de-toxify the liver and gall bladder as well as getting rid of gallstones if there are any, the following regime is helpful:

1. For about 1 week, eliminate fatty foods and starchy foods. Eat primarily vegetables, a few whole grains, and perhaps some fish if you desire it.
2. Before going to sleep, make a drink with 2 t. psyllium seeds and 1 T. of bentonite. These can be mixed in herb tea or a little fruit juice if your system can tolerate it. Have another drink in the morning as well. The psyllium and bentonite will cleanse the small intestine, ridding it of candida and yeast, as well as preparing the body for the liver flush.
3. The day you are going to do the flush, eat a light lunch, salad or vegetables.
4. Three hours later, take 2 t. or 3 capsules of di-sodium phosphate mixed in herb tea or hot water. You may add a little fruit juice for flavor.
5. Repeat this 2 hours later.
6. For dinner, have some vegetable juice or vegetable broth.
7. Before going to sleep, take 1/2 cup olive oil blended with the juice of 1 lemon.
8. Go immediately to bed, lie on your right side with your right knee pulled close to your chest for 30 minutes.

The next morning you may find small gallstone-type objects in the stool which are light to dark green in color. They are irregular in shape, gelatinous in texture, and vary in size from grape seeds to cherry seeds. If you do find these, repeat this procedure in two weeks. If you don't find these, you still may want to repeat this procedure every six months or yearly.

A simple way to cleanse the liver is to take about 1/4 or 1/3 cup of olive oil mixed with the juice of 1/2 a lemon upon rising, a few times a week. Wait at least an hour before eating, although herb teas may be drunk.

Drinking alcohol of any kind, using drugs including prescription medicines, being around strong chemical smells from detergents and household cleansers as well as airborne pollutants, all contribute to liver toxicity. People who have strong allergic reactions always have a toxic liver. If the liver is clean and doing its work, it will eliminate most of the allergens from the bloodstream and strong histamine reactions such as sneezing, runny eyes and nose, and skin irritations will not occur.

The *kidneys* are the organs controlling elimination in the body; they are also responsible for maintaining the acid-alkaline balance along with the respiratory system. The kidneys filter the entire volume of blood in the body 60 times a day. If the kidneys are too busy eliminating toxic material such as heavy metals or chemicals, they cannot fulfill their other functions. It is important to keep the kidneys cleansed. This can be done periodically by drinking parsley tea upon rising, a couple of cups of parsley tea a few times a week. Parsley tea is made by simmering a small bunch of parsley in a few cups of purified water. Another way to cleanse the kidneys is with high doses of Vitamin C. Utilizing a buffered powdered Vitamin C and using 1 t. about 2 or 3 times a day can help to clear out toxicity.

When the liver and kidneys are very toxic, skin problems often arise. Skin eruptions are a sign that the body needs to eliminate. In addition to cleansing the organs mentioned above, saunas and steam baths are excellent methods of cleansing the skin, especially in the winter months when we don't normally perspire. The sweat lodge, used by many traditional cultures, is an excellent way of purifying the body along with the spirit.

Certain foods and herbs are also important in cleansing the body. *Mucilaginous* foods and herbs lubricate the walls of the colon and aid elimination. Mucilaginous foods include psyllium husks, flax seeds, and chia seeds. These can be ground up and added to cereal, sprinkled on salads or soups, or taken mixed with water or herb teas. Herbs that are mucilaginous include aloe vera juice, slippery elm, and comfrey leaf.

Including *fermented foods* in the diet is also important as an aid to elimination and to promote growth of healthy intestinal bacteria. Yogurt and kefir are among these foods but are generally made from cow's milk which produces a type of *pathogenic mucus* (not the lubricating mucus in the mucosa) that propagates germs and bacteria. However, goat's milk yogurt is available. Seed yogurts and cheeses can also be made from sesame seeds, sunflower seeds, and other seeds. Fermented foods made from soybeans include *miso* (a soup broth or base) and *tamari* (soy sauce). One should be careful, however, in utilizing these foods as they are very high in sodium and may upset the acid/alkaline balance. Yellow and white misos are lower in sodium. Other fermented foods include sauerkraut and *kim chee* (an Oriental spicy mix of cabbage and red peppers that has been fermented).

CLEANSING BATHS

Therapeutic bathing is most important in de-toxifying the body. Four thousand years ago, the Egyptians developed bathing into a high art, using mineral salts and scented oils. Most of us are exposed to environmental radiation, dental x-rays, and additional radiation from air travel. Dr. Hazel Parcells, who lived to the age of 105 in northern New Mexico, worked for many years to discover methods of removing pesticides and irradiation from foods as well as from our bodies. She developed and used these formulas for many years.

For radiation and general toxicity, bathe several times a week with the following formula; when your body is more balanced, continue to bathe weekly with this formula. Dissolve one pound of sea salt and one pound of baking soda in a tub of water as hot as can be tolerated. Stay in the bathtub as long as you can until the water has cooled and do not shower for eight hours following the bath.

If you have been exposed to heavy metals such as aluminum or carbon monoxide or pesticide sprays, you may experience decreased energy, shortness of breath, or impaired balance. The following bath will help. Add a cup of regular brand Clorox to a tub of water as hot as you can tolerate. Stay in the bath until the water has cooled and do not shower for eight hours.

If you are suffering from general muscle aches brought about by physical exertion or mental or emotional stress, add two cups of apple cider vinegar to a tub of water as hot as can be tolerated. Stay in the bath as long as you can until the water has cooled and do not shower for eight hours.

Cleansing baths will make internal cleansing of the colon, liver, and kidneys more effective and help in boosting the immune system.

CHAPTER 8:
METABOLISM AND DIET

While many harmful substances and poisons are easy to identify—arsenic for example—some foods which are good for certain people, may be totally inappropriate for others. For example, some people thrive on a diet that includes beans and legumes; others would suffer from chronic gas. Some people can tolerate breads and baked goods made from wheat; others develop mucus, become tired, or have an allergic reaction. How do we determine what is harmful or beneficial for each of us?

In our daily observation of people, we experience many physical types—those whose bodies are tall and thin, others who are shorter or heavier, some whose complexions are ruddy, others who are pale or sallow. We also see those who are nervous, tense, and underweight as well as those who are more relaxed with a heavier frame. All of these qualities are due to *individual metabolism*.

Metabolism is the function of maintaining life; it is the total exchange of energy with the environment, an exchange involving food, water, air, light, and heat. How each of us uses these raw materials to maintain life differs from one person to another.

In Western medicine and physiology, we speak of metabolic constitutions being determined by the dominance of the sympathetic or parasympathetic nervous systems. *Sympathetic dominance* leads to action-oriented, hyperactive, tense, underweight individuals. They often have problems with constipation; dryness around the mouth, eyes and nose; cold extremities; and adrenal exhaustion. *Parasympathetics* tend to be slower and less active, fall asleep more easily, often have ruddy complexions, and rely more on intuition than reason. Sympathetic dominance is characterized by slow oxidation and digestion because most of the nervous impulses are going to the energy-producing glands. Parasympathetic dominance, on the other hand, has faster oxidation and digestion; these individuals are prone to diarrhea, stomach and intestinal problems, and low blood sugar because they metabolize so fast.

In Ayurvedic medicine, the ancient Hindu system of healing, individuals are categorized by the predominating *dosha* or element—*Vata*, or Air, *Pitta*, or Fire, *Kapha*, or Water. Vata types are very mental, tend to be thin and wiry, and often have problems with constipation and digestion; they are fairly slow oxidizers. Pitta types are fiery, active and energetic, producing a good amount of bile and breaking down foods easily; they are fast oxidizers and are more prone to diarrhea and digestive problems relating to the liver. Kapha types are more emotional, move slowly, and often are heavier due to excess water they carry in their bodies; they are very slow oxidizers.

The various types resulting from sympathetic or parasympathetic dominance have been organized into a system of ten *metabolic types* by Dr. William Donald Kelley, a dentist who cured himself of liver and pancreatic cancer (see *One Answer to Cancer*, The Kelley Foundation, 1974). Kelley found that the diet and supplements that helped him did not work for his wife when she was ill with cancer. In discovering a totally different diet for his wife, Kelley stumbled on an idea that led him to investigate these two branches of the autonomic nervous system.

The autonomic nervous system which regulates metabolism controls involuntary metabolic actions such as heartbeat and digestion. Dr. Kelley found that most people are neurologically influenced more strongly by either the 'accelerator" (sympathetic) or 'decelerator" (parasympathetic) branch of the autonomic nervous system. Some people may be healthy with 'accelerating" or 'decelerating" nerve stimulation, while others may be just as healthy with 'balanced" stimulation.

The varying degrees of nerve stimulation mean that one's glands and organs function differently. This affects our chemical and hormonal output, which in turn affects personality traits and behavioral patterns as well as physiological characteristics.

Once the metabolic type is determined, the proper nutrients for an individual can be recommended in the form of foods and nutritional supplements. Dr. Kelley identified ten metabolic types ranging from those with pure sympathetic dominance to those with pure parasympathetic dominance. Most people fall in between the two extremes.

Individuals whose sympathetic nervous system is more dominant receive less nerve stimulation in the digestive organs and more in the energy-producing glands. Those dominated by the parasympathetic branch receive more nerve stimulation to the digestive organs and less in the energy-producing glands. Many individuals are balanced; they are neither sympathetically nor parasympathetically dominated.

Individuals dominated by the sympathetic nervous system are often prone to anxiety, nervous strain, and irritability. Parasympathetics tend to have a slow metabolism, indicating that they oxidize blood sugar rapidly and, therefore, have low blood sugar. Those with sympathetic dominance experience food as a heavy feeling in the stomach. Their 'fast metabolism" emphasizes the *catabolic* aspect of metabolism which breaks down complex substances into simpler ones. Catabolic processes take place in the absence of oxygen, so the sympathetic oxidizes blood sugar slowly. They have a more acidic body chemistry and do better with alkaline foods such as vegetables. Since the food stays with them so long, they need to eat lightly as they can easily build up waste products in the digestive tract. Parasympathetics and more balanced types can eat more at one sitting. The slow metabolism of the parasympathetic emphasizes the *anabolic* aspect of metabolism, which synthesizes complex substances from simple ones. Anabolic processes are aerobic (take place in the presence of oxygen), so the parasympathetic oxidizes blood sugar rapidly.

How does one determine whether her/his metabolism is dominated more by the sympathetic or parasympathetic system?

Sympathetic	Parasympathetic
rarely craves sugar	craves sugar frequently
eats small meals often	can eat larger meals
prefers vegetables	often desires meat and heavy proteins
wakes up easily	difficulty getting out of bed
active during the day	often lethargic and sluggish
worries a lot	more relaxed and less anxious
likes exercise	dislikes exercise
makes decisions easily	often has difficulty making decisions
good concentration	poor concentration
acts more on reason	acts more on intuition

These characteristics are the extreme of each type; most of us are combinations of the two, though we often have one system that is more dominant.

ACID/ALKALINE BALANCE

The acid/alkaline balance is a subtle issue since there are many layers of pH in the body. The pH number measures acidity and alkalinity, with 7 being neutral, less than 7 being acid, more than 7 being alkaline. However, the body has many different pH values—the skin and saliva are slightly acid; the stomach is much more acid; the small intestine is alkaline; the large intestine is slightly acid; blood and cells are slightly alkaline, and urine is somewhat acid. The blood needs to preserve its alkalinity and buffers the acids with calcium.

Dr. William Kelley explains that in a 24-hour period the body has two peak periods of alkalinity. These are times of cellular repair, lasting 2 1/2 to 3 hours, peaking about 3:30 AM and 2:30 PM. The fluctuations between these cycles is known as the acid/alkaline cycle.

Certain times of the day one would be more alkaline than others; this would be dependent on emotional and mental states and not just our diet. Highly sensitive and psychic individuals tend to be more acid as do many artistic people.

Some individuals need more alkaline foods and less acid ones. They often manifest symptoms that are indicative of this. Arthritis, ulcers, hyperactivity, and often allergies point to the need for more alkaline foods.

There are many theories of acid and alkaline for foods. My own experience comes from many years of working with clients in the healing arena and understanding their bodies through both dowsing and kinesiology. People with herpes, candida, hypoglycemia, diabetes, digestive problems, and many allergies need to eliminate fruits and acid foods, along with sugar, for a considerable time period.

The following foods are categorized as acids: all fruits and fruit juices, sugars, tomatoes, spinach (high in oxalic acid), green pepper, chocolate, black teas (high in tannic acids), coffee, vinegar, and nutritional yeast (many people are allergic to this).

METABOLIC CONSTITUTIONS AS SEEN THROUGH AYURVEDIC MEDICINE

In order to compare the differing metabolisms, we need to understand the meaning of each of the three doshas. *Vata* is the principle of *kinetic energy* in the body; it is concerned with the nervous system and controls all body movements. *Kapha* is the principle of *potential energy*, which controls body stability and lubrication. *Pitta* controls the body's *balance* of kinetic and potential energies; the enzyme system and endocrine system are Pitta's territory.

At the cellular level, Vata moves nutrients into, and wastes out of, cells. Pitta digests nutrients to provide for cellular function, and the cell's structure is governed by Kapha. In the digestive tract, Vata assimilates nutrients and expels wastes, and Kapha controls the secretions that lubricate and protect the digestive organs.

Vata is not gas, but increased Vata causes increased gas. Kapha is not mucus, but it is the force that is projected in the body and causes mucus to arise. Pitta is not bile, but it is the force that causes bile to be produced.

Most people are combinations of these types and are Vata-Pitta, Pitta-Kapha, or Vata-Kapha.

In terms of food, Vata types have irregular appetites—they often suffer from constipation. Pitta types love to eat; they usually digest well, have loose stools, and are rarely constipated. Kapha types can become attached to food as a means of emotional fulfillment. Vata types do better with three or four small meals a day; they often need to snack in between, but not more than every 2 hours (the time it takes for food to digest). Pitta types should eat three meals daily with 4–6 hours between them. Kapha types should eat only twice a day with a 6-hour gap between meals.

Vata types require more cooked food than Pitta or Kapha types. Pitta or Pitta-Kapha can handle more raw foods because they have the digestive fire to break them down. Vata people do best on one-pot meals like soups, stews, or casseroles because they are easier to digest than individual foods.

Vata	Pitta	Kapha
rarely craves sweets	on occasion craves sweets	craves sweets
lots of nervous energy	good physical energy	often lethargic
insomnia and restless	sleeps well	sleeps well
wakes up easily	wakes up easily	difficulty waking
likes exercise	often overdoes exercise	dislikes exercise
logical	logical and intuitive	intuitive
irregular appetite	loves to eat	food emotionally fulfilling

DIET

Diet in the Ayurvedic system is based on six tastes:

1. Sweet is cooling, heavy, and oily. It increases Kapha, decreases Pitta and Vata.
2. Sour is heating, heavy, and oily. It encourages elimination of wastes, lessens spasms and tremors, and improves appetite and digestion.
3. Salty is heating, heavy, and oily. It eliminates wastes, cleans the body, and increases digestive capacity and appetite as well as softening and loosening tissues.
4. Pungent (hot and spicy like chili peppers) is heating, light, and dry. It flushes all secretions from the body and improves the appetite. It increases Pitta and Vata, and decreases Kapha.

5. Bitter is cooling, light, and dry. It purifies and dries all secretions, increases appetite and controls skin disease and fevers. It increases Vata, decreases Pitta and Kapha.

6. Astringent (makes one's mouth pucker) is cooling, light, and dry. It reduces secretions and purifies and constricts part of the body. It increases Vata, decreases Pitta and Kapha.

Foods for Vata Constitutions

Sweet, sour, and salty foods are good for Vata constitutions; bitter, pungent, and astringent are less desirable because they dry out the system. In terms of grains, well-cooked rice and oats are excellent. Cooked buckwheat, millet, and rye are heating and therefore good. Yeasted bread is not so good because the fermentation creates gas in Vata types. Freshly cooked grains are better since bread is dried out by baking.

Cooked vegetables are preferable to raw vegetables. Rough, hard vegetables like celery are better digested as juice. Salads of lettuce, parsley, cilantro or sprouts may be eaten on occasion with a good oily salad dressing like olive oil. Tomatoes are not good raw but infrequently may be used cooked where the skins and seeds are removed.

Some fruits are good such as papaya, peaches, cherries, and some melons like cantaloupe. Grapes, plums, strawberries, and watermelon are too acidic. Dried fruits should be reconstituted with water. Apples and pears are best baked. Ripe bananas are good because they are soothing to the intestine and are helpful for constipation.

Vata is considered the only type who needs animal foods because they need the complete proteins. Too much animal flesh weakens the digestive tract, however. Eggs, fresh fish, chicken, turkey, and liver may be used (providing they are organic) Soured-milk products, such as yogurt or kefir, may be used since they aid digestion. Eggs should be scrambled with yogurt or poached; fried eggs are not good.

Legumes are difficult to digest and their metabolic by-product is nitrogen, which is a gas that increases Vata. Mung beans are the lightest to digest. Legumes may be cooked with turmeric, cumin, or coriander seeds to kindle digestive fire. They also may be cooked with ginger or garlic. If legumes are soaked for an hour and the water thrown away, they tend to produce less gas. Splitting peas and lentils makes them more digestible because more of the surface is exposed while cooking.

Almonds are the best nuts, but they should be soaked overnight and their skins peeled. Other seeds and nuts should be made into nut milks or butters so they will not be too concentrated. Overconcentrated foods resist penetration by digestive juices.

All oils are good for Vata types, especially olive, almond, and sesame. Coconut and sesame oils can be used for the hair and skin.

Some sweets reduce Vata; barley malt syrup, rice syrup, molasses or honey may be used. The overuse of sweets increases Vata.

All spices, especially garlic and ginger, can be ingested by Vata types in small amounts. Vata types tend to overuse hot spices to improve digestion so they should be used with care. Cayenne, cardamom, curry, and turmeric are warming and aid digestion. Fennel, dill, and anise are good for gas.

Foods for Pitta Constitutions

Pitta types should avoid sour, salty, and pungent, but should use sweet, bitter, and astringent. Meat, alcohol, and salt should especially be avoided because they increase heat and aggressiveness. Grains, vegetables, and some fruit should form the majority of the Pitta diet.

Barley is the best grain for Pitta types because it is cooling and drying and helps reduce excess stomach acid. Rice and oats are also good. Buckwheat, millet, and rye may be too heating, but can be used sometimes. Yeasted bread is not good because of the sourness produced during fermentation, but unyeasted bread is fine.

Most vegetables are beneficial for Pitta types, except sour vegetables such as tomatoes, and pungent vegetables such as radishes. Beets, carrots, and daikon radish are good for the liver.

Pitta types should eat sweet fruit and avoid sour fruit like oranges, lemons, limes, pineapples, and pomegranates.

Flesh food is not recommended for Pitta people, but fresh fish, as well as turkey or chicken on occasion are okay.

Legumes should be eaten sparingly because of their acidity, but mung beans, tofu, black lentils, split peas, and chickpeas (red and yellow) are fine. Lentils are too warming.

Nuts and seeds are too hot and oily, except for coconut milk, which is cooling.

Sweet dairy products like milk, ghee, and unsalted cheeses are best.

Sweets can be better handled by Pitta types than other types. However, molasses is heating, and honey can be heating if it is overused. Only cooling spices such as fennel and dill should be used; cardamom, cinnamon, and turmeric should be used rarely.

Foods for Kapha Constitutions

Kapha types need to concentrate on bitter, pungent, and astringent foods to invigorate their body and mind and should avoid sweet, sour, and salty tastes. Fat greasy foods and dairy products are the worst foods for these people. They need grains less than the other types, but hot drying grains like buckwheat and millet work best for them. Barley, rice, and corn are also beneficial. Breads are best toasted or dried out.

All vegetables are good for Kapha types, except tomatoes and very sour vegetables. Leafy greens are preferable to root vegetables. Steamed and stir-fried vegetables are easier to digest than raw, though raw vegetables may be eaten on occasion.

Very sweet and very sour fruits should be avoided as well as any fruits that are extremely juicy. Dried fruits are good, such as mangoes, apples, pears, apricots, and peaches.

Kapha people rarely need any flesh foods, but they may eat fresh fish, eggs, or broiled poultry. Legumes are better for Kapha types than flesh foods, but they do not need much protein. Heavy legumes like soybeans, kidney beans, and black lentils should be avoided.

Nuts and seeds also should be avoided since they are too oily. The same goes for most oils, except for flax, olive, almond, or safflower oils on occasion.

Dairy products are not particularly good, as previously mentioned, though goat's milk products are better than cow's milk.

Sweets should be avoided since they increase Kapha. All spices may be used except salt; ginger and garlic are especially good.

Other Types

Vata-Pitta types should follow a Vata-controlling diet in fall and winter and a Pitta-controlling diet in spring and summer when Pitta is stronger. They should especially avoid spicy, pungent food.

Pitta-Kapha types should use a Pitta-controlling diet from late spring through early fall and a Kapha-controlling diet from late fall through early spring. Bitter and astringent tastes are best for these types.

Vata-Kaphas should control Vata in summer and fall and Kapha in winter and spring. Since both Vata and Kapha are cold and need heat, they should use sour, salty, and pungent tastes rather than sweet, bitter, and astringent tastes.

These are all general guidelines from the Ayurvedic system and they must be tailored to individual taste and temperament. Though individuals may be typed metabolically, there are many differences within each type and many systems of diet.

CHAPTER 9: DIETARY REGIMENS

M any answers have been given to the question, "What foods are best for me? Which foods should I avoid?" This chapter covers several of the major dietary approaches.

All of these regimens feature natural foods, but there are many types of diets within the spectrum of natural dietary regimens. A nonvegetarian natural diet may include fish, organic poultry, and some other organic meats. Lacto-vegetarians include dairy products and eggs in their diet. Vegans eat no dairy products or eggs; their protein sources are nuts, seeds, tofu (soybean curd), and legumes.

Another distinction in vegetarian diets is those that recommend mostly raw foods and those that use mostly cooked foods. Raw food diets have been popular in warm climates where there is an abundance of fresh fruits and vegetables, and body temperature is able to maintain itself without warm, cooked foods. They also are utilized by those who are on a cleansing diet or preparing for a fast, or those who have a serious illness and need to eat a light diet and eliminate protein.

RAW FOODS

Enthusiasts of raw food diets say that enzymes are killed in the cooking process thus making nutrients less available. They do not believe in eating grains because grains form mucus in the system which they claim may reduce the entrance of oxygen into the lungs.

Grains contain a high concentration of starch and mineral salts. When subjected to heat, these minerals are rendered insoluble and may be deposited in body tissues. In addition, unsprouted grains are acid-forming in the body. To replace cooked grains, cooked tubers or squash are recommended.

Foods should not be eaten cold either. They should be taken out of the refrigerator and allowed to soak in the sun to absorb solar radiation. Some researchers believe that raw food enzymes continue to work in conjunction with digestive enzymes in the stomach. In the intestines, vegetable enzymes help to detoxify intestinal flora as well as to normalize bacteria in the colon. This reduces the number of disease-producing bacteria.

Dr. Ann Wigmore has become famous for her healing of disease through the use of raw foods and wheat grass juice. She set up the Hippocrates Health Institute (there is one in Boston and one in San Diego) where patients learn how to grow sprouts and to juice raw foods. (She has several books out, including *Why Suffer*, which delineates the discovery of wheat grass and its effect on health). Many people attribute their ability to heal themselves of cancer and other life-threatening diseases to a raw-food diet with lots of vegetable juices.

MACROBIOTICS

The Macrobiotic Diet was developed by the Japanese philosopher George Ohsawa. (*Macro* means "large" or "great," and *bios* means "life.") Ohsawa felt that with a good diet we could experience a deep and fulfilling life. In addition to being a preventive diet to maintain health, Macrobiotics has been used therapeutically for those who are seriously ill.

In Macrobiotics, food is considered not just for its physical effect but for its mental and spiritual effect. Each piece of food is treated as a spiritual manifestation and should not be wasted in the process of preparing and cooking. Before eating, prayers should be offered to nature and the Universe, which have given us this food. While eating, it is important to chew each particle of food thoroughly in order to spiritualize it and to reflect on the harmony of the universe.

Macrobiotics classifies foods according to *yin* and *yang*.

Yin	Yang
grows in hot climate	grows in cold climate
contains more water	is more dry
fruits and leaves	stems, roots, and seeds
high above the ground	below the ground
acid reaction in the body	alkaline reaction in the body
hot, aromatic foods	salty, sour foods

During the winter, the climate is cold and damp (yin); thus, the energy descends into the roots, leaves die, the sap goes to the roots, and the vitality of the plant becomes more yang. Plants that grow in late autumn and winter are more dry and have more vitality; they can also be kept a long time without spoiling. Examples are root vegetables such as carrots, turnips, parsnips, and cabbages. The weather becomes more hot and dry (yang). Summer vegetables are more watery and perishable; they need to be stored in a cool place. Fruits ripen in late summer; they are watery and sweet and develop higher above the ground. Foods which grow in hot tropical climates are more yin, whereas foods which grow in northern climates are more yang.

Constituents of the Macrobiotic Diet

1. Grains are the staple of the diet: brown rice, buckwheat, millet, rye, oats, barley, corn, and whole wheat form 50–60% of the diet used as whole grains, cereals, and breads.
2. Legumes and seeds form 10–15% of the diet and can be used at every meal in combination with grains.
3. Twenty to thirty percent of the diet is land and sea vegetables, including soups. About two-thirds of these are cooked, and about one-third is raw in the form of salads. Potatoes (including sweet potatoes and yams), tomatoes, eggplant, avocado, and other tropical vegetables are avoided. Seaweeds such as dulse, kombu, wakame, hijiki, arame, and agar-agar are used.
4. Less than 15% animal food is used—primarily white meat fish and seafood.
5. Fruits and nuts are used in small amounts; a fruit dessert is served on occasion if the fruit is growing in the same climatic zone.
6. Fermented food is used in small amounts to provide enzymes and bacteria. These include vegetable-based fermented foods such as miso, tamari, soy sauce, sauerkraut, and other pickles.
7. Beverages predominantly made of non-aromatic herbs like bancha twig tea, mu tea, dandelion tea, burdock tea, or cereal grains are used. These should be taken as the last part of the meal or separately.
8. Sweets are avoided, except rice syrup, barley malt syrup, or other syrups processed from grains. These are used on occasion.

The diet also prescribes a definite order for eating. Whole grains, legumes, and seeds can be eaten throughout the meal. Soups are eaten first, then vegetables, and then vegetable salads or pickles. Fish is often included with the vegetables. Fruit, nuts, and beverages are used at the end of the meal and consumed alone. Seasonings include soy sauce, unrefined sea salt, and vegetable oil. Tropical spices and aromatic herbs are avoided.

Some people find the Macrobiotic Diet too heavy because of its emphasis on grains and legumes. Certain body types have difficulty digesting grains and are better off eating grains only once a day, preferably in the morning. In the

Ayurvedic system, Vata types, generally thin, airy, and mental people, do not have the enzymes to break down carbohydrates. They do need more protein than other types, however. Kapha types, heavy body types whose bodies seem to be filled with water, may also need a lighter diet since they produce a lot of mucus. They often do better with a light breakfast (vegetables or fruit) rather than a grain breakfast.

The Macrobiotic Diet and certain fasts (combinations of brown rice with vegetables and some fish) have proved very healing for those with many serious ailments. Dr. Anthony Sattilaro, in Philadelphia, healed himself of cancer through the use of the Macrobiotic Diet and its philosophy. Author of *Recalled by Life*, he is one of macrobiotics' strongest advocates.

OTHER DIETS

More moderate diets than those consisting of raw foods, or Macrobiotics work for most people. Whole grains are very grounding and contain most of the B-complex vitamins and other nutrients. Most people respond well to eating a whole-grain cereal or the whole grains themselves in the morning. This is because the grain is a complex carbohydrate and takes about eight hours to break down in the body. This process of breaking down helps keep the blood sugar up. Whole-grain breads are okay but do not have as many nutrients as the grains themselves. Vegetables may be added to the grain; proteins like eggs, tofu, or fish may also be eaten with the grain for a more substantial meal. Those with low blood sugar do well if they have some protein in the morning. As was mentioned previously, certain metabolic types that tend to accumulate mucus function better on a very light breakfast of vegetable juices or cooked vegetables or fruit.

The midday meal should be the largest meal, but this is not always possible for many people who work and bring their food to the office or have to eat at a restaurant. Midday meals should include some vegetables, whether in the form of soups, steamed, or raw in salads. Certain metabolic types and those with low blood sugar benefit from good protein at their midday meal. This may be eggs or fish (if they are eaten) or a soy product like tofu. (Dairy products like cheese tend to form a lot of mucus and are responsible for many allergic conditions. They should be used primarily in the form of soured-milk products like yogurts, kefir, buttermilk, acidophilis cottage cheese, or a small amount of goat milk cheese.) Some people need heavier foods at midday—a grain or bread, or root vegetables like potatoes or squash.

What one has for dinner depends on what was eaten for the midday meal. Ideally, dinner should be the lightest meal since one goes to sleep several hours afterwards. Digestive enzymes work best at midday; that is when our fire is at its greatest (the internal fire creates the enzymes that break down food).

Steamed or raw vegetables should be included at dinner with some protein, grain, or root vegetable. Heavy carbohydrates such as pasta, beans, and breads should be avoided, as well as heavy proteins and fatty foods like meats and dairy products. Fruits should be eaten separately as snacks in between meals unless it is an all-fruit meal. Fruits can be very acid and are difficult to digest with other foods. Beverages are best after a meal as well, except for vegetable juices which may be drunk before a meal. Herbal teas and grain beverages should be served a short while after eating since the liquids wash away the digestive enzymes.

Alcoholic beverages drunk with meals also have an acidic effect and may interfere with the digestive process. Alcoholic beverages in general are not particularly good for the liver and may interfere with bile production. Certain foods like vinegar, nutritional yeast, cranberries, raw green pepper, and tomatoes are very acidic and should be avoided. (Tomatoes may be used on occasion in a cooked sauce.)

Wheat products form a lot of mucus, and many people are allergic to them. Rye bread, rice bread, and other wheatless breads such as millet bread may be substituted. Rye flour, rice flour, buckwheat flour, millet flour, barley flour, and oat flour may be used in baking instead of wholewheat flour.

A balanced diet includes whole grains at least once a day; vegetables, raw or cooked, twice a day; protein, once a day; and fruit, for those whose bodies are not too acid, as a snack. If sweets are used, they should be made with honey, barley malt syrup, or rice syrup. Those with low blood sugar do best with the syrups made from grains because they have more complex carbohydrates. There are many cookies and candy bars where these syrups are used; many are also fruit-juice sweetened.

For those who have certain food addictions and cravings, there are ways to balance the body and substitute healthier foods. Many people are used to drinking coffee in the morning and at other times of the day to wake them up. The caffeine in coffee is a stimulant to the nervous system and is also very acidic but it can make one very wired without really increasing vitality or energy. Herbs like gotu-kola or fo-ti which do, in fact, increase adrenal energy, can be used instead. If one likes the taste of coffee, there are grain beverages such as Roma, Cafix, or Pero, which are coffee substitutes.

Many people crave sugar, especially mid-afternoon when their energy drops. Usually if they eat a substantial breakfast with a cooked whole-grain product, blood sugar remains higher. Utilizing a pancreas glandular supplement after meals, or an amino acid capsule, or digestive enzymes can help to stabilize the blood sugar. However, it is a good idea to have a mid-afternoon snack like a piece of fresh fruit, raw vegetables, or some nuts or seeds. If one wants something sweet, cookies or a candy bar with natural sweetening may be eaten on occasion.

Variety in foods is a good principle to abide by in order to obtain nutrients and to avoid allergies. Eating a different grain every morning is a way to vary breakfasts. Using different vegetables for lunch and dinner and alternating the type of protein is another way to create variety. The way foods are served may also add nutrition. Foods in combination with certain proteins produce essential amino acids; for example, adding seeds or tofu to a grain dish.

Diet includes much more than the food itself. Diet includes the type of food we buy. Is it organic, or does it have chemical additives? Where was it grown? What kind of store was it bought in? All these factors affect the vibrational quality of the food we eat. How we prepare the food also affects it; if we are feeling angry or upset, it might be better to have a snack and wait until we feel more balanced. In fact, we will take in those angry vibrations with our food; this often is why people get indigestion. It is better to eat meals slowly in a relaxed atmosphere than at one's desk or while driving to and from places. Food eaten in a relaxed atmosphere will be much more healing to our bodies than food—no matter how high the quality—eaten on the run.

We are what we eat has been a much-overused statement. As spiritual beings, we know we are more than our food intake. Perhaps we could change the statement to "We are *how* we eat." How we eat reflects how we nurture ourselves and each other, and ultimately, how we treat our environment.

CHAPTER 10: HERBOLOGY

Paracelsus warned that drugs used to cure illnesses can hurt the body. Many conventional drugs, which often work by simply suppressing symptoms or by creating chemical changes in an imblanced body to simulate the action of a balanced body, do nothing to correct the underlying problems, and often exacerbate imbalances. In contrast, herbs have three major functions, each of which supports the body's ability to heal itself. First, they can eliminate toxins from the body and cleanse it; such herbs include blood purifiers, diuretics, and laxatives. Second, they can help the body heal itself by building or maintaining the body. Third, some herbs have a toning affect on the whole body or certain organs; they strengthen or improve that organ or system as well as improve the blood flow.

From earliest times we have been surrounded with plants, and by observing where these plants grow and experimenting with the different parts of them—the flowers, roots, leaves—we have been able to heal ourselves of many ailments.

Utilizing plant medicine is such a strong form of healing because it connects us with our environment, with Gaia, with the living Earth. Plants were placed in our environment so that we might *relate* to them; this relationship includes touching, smelling, and utilizing them for their medicinal properties in teas, tinctures, poultices, and salves. Plants are our teachers; by observing them and ingesting them when appropriate, we may become attuned to many spiritual and metaphysical truths.

Herbs can be used both internally in the form of teas, tinctures, and capsules and externally as salves, ointments, and poultices. The first pharmacies made their medicines exclusively from herbs. Many of these are still around as cough syrups and cough drops from horehound and wild cherry bark, liniments from wintergreen and eucalyptus. Some medications used in treating serious diseases are also derived from herbs; an example would be digitalis, used for heart conditions, which comes from the herb foxglove. Certain herbs have a toning effect on specific organs or systems in the body. Dandelion root tones the liver and pancreas; comfrey root, the lungs and large intestine.

Herbs have many properties which combine to make them strong medicines. First is their *smell* or scent—the aroma of an herb can produce an effect before it is even ingested. The smell of peppermint, for example, begins to soothe and stimulate the digestive tract before the tea is drunk. *Aromatherapy* is a branch of herbology where the herbs are used specifically for their scents. The *taste* of herbs is another factor: sour tastes work on detoxifying; salty tastes influence the water balance; sweet tastes are nutritive; bitter tastes fight inflammation and cleanse the liver; pungent tastes open the respiratory tract and skin.

There are a number of herbal therapies that are used to treat different types of disease. In the course of a disease, several of these therapies might be appropriate, depending on the energy level of individuals and the changes in their bodies at the time.

DETOXIFYING OR CLEANSING

Detoxifying includes sweating, vomiting, and purging. *Sweating* is used to treat diseases such as cold, flu, and fevers. Stimulating diaphoretic (herbs used to induce sweating) teas provide heat and increase circulation; they treat weaknesses in the internal organs. (Stomach and bowels should be emptied before ingesting through fasting, an enema, or a colonic irrigation.) Teas made from ginger, cayenne, Chinese cinnamon (cassia bark), and peppermint are in this category. Relaxing diaphoretic teas such as catnip, spearmint, skullcap, or lemon balm treat ailments in which the pores of the skin are closed and the energy has retreated from the surface. In addition, a hot bath or sauna should be taken after which one bundles up with warm blankets to promote sweating.

Emetic herbs induce *vomiting* and are used after eating poor food combinations to alleviate food poisoning. Ipecac is an herbal syrup which is a useful emetic. Other herbs may also be used, but caution should be exercised in using emetics since overuse tends to weaken the individual and deplete the vitality.

Purging through herbal laxatives may be helpful in treating excess toxins or constipation. One should be extremely careful, however, in using herbal laxatives as they often force food through the intestinal canal too quickly. They also deplete energy. Dietary changes and the addition of mucilaginous foods and herbs should be used to improve elimination. Colonic irrigations and enemas help cleansing and detoxifying.

Mild herbs like slippery elm, marshmallow root, and comfrey are soothing to the intestinal mucus and may be readily used. Aloe vera juice may also be utilized; it is beneficial to the mucous linings and helps to cleanse the colon. Ground psyllium seed, flaxseed, and chia seeds may be added to grains or other foods. These are bulk laxatives which increase bulk in the intestinal tract, thus aiding peristalsis. Other herbs stimulate bile secretions which also have a laxative effect. Herbs in this category include Oregon grape root, wild yam, and rhubarb.

BLOOD PURIFYING

Most diseases can be eliminated through "purifying the blood" and neutralizing excess acidity in the body. The concept of "blood purifying" is an old one in Western folk medicine; it is not a scientific concept. The idea is that the system can become toxic, poisoned, stagnant, and inflamed. When the bloodstream is "toxic," it indicates that the lymphatics are stagnant, being glutted with waste materials; the liver is not able to detoxify substances entering the organism from the intestinal blood supply, which is rich with food and toxic wastes; the kidneys are not able to remove uric acid (wastes) from the blood. This stagnation and intoxification results in local tissue irritation, redness, burning, swelling, and skin rashes. Herbs that work on the liver, lymphatics, and kidneys are called "blood purifiers" or *alteratives.*

Some "blood purifiers" include echinacea root, chaparral, red clover, sarsaparilla root, sassafras, cleavers, nettles, burdock root, yellow dock root, and goldenseal.

TRANQUILIZING

Tranquilizing herbs are used when there are conditions of restlessness, nervousness, or spasms accompanying illness. There are three types of tranquilizers: demulcents, nervines, and anti-spasmodics.

Demulcents lubricate the gastrointestinal tract and other mucous linings of our bodies. Herbs such as slippery elm, comfrey root and leaf, and marshmallow root are mucilaginous and serve to lubricate bones and joints as well. *Nervines* or nerve tonics help to balance out the nervous system. These include chamomile, catnip, skullcap, wood betony, hops, spearmint, vervain, and valerian. *Anti-spasmodics* relax tension in muscles; they also help to relieve pain due to tension. Herbal anti-spasmodics include lobelia, hops, vervain, and valerian.

STIMULATING

Herbal *stimulants* add to the vitality of the various organs by increasing metabolism, circulation, and the breaking up of obstructions in the body. Disease often results through blockages in the blood, lymph system, and digestive tract.

When there is decreased vitality, chills, sluggishness, weak digestion, lower back pain, and the beginning of conditions such as colds and flus, stimulation therapy is helpful. Stimulants may be used alone or added to other herbs to increase their activity and help promote circulation and detoxification. For poor digestion, some of the culinary herbs are mild stimulants. These include cardamom, cloves, cumin, coriander, and cayenne. Ginger is another good stimulant and is often used as a tea, in cooking, or as a compress externally.

TONING

Toning or tonification therapy is used to strengthen the blood, various organs, and the vitality of the body. It is used after acute diseases, during chronic disease to build the energy for detoxification, and to recover from injuries, childbirth, and surgeries.

After acute diseases, foods such as vegetable juices, broths, and other foods high in minerals and vitamins should be used (seaweeds, wheat grass juice, and sprouts). Mild herbal tonics, such as comfrey, nettles, alfalfa, plantain, chickweed, and watercress, may be used in salads or teas. Later, stronger tonics such as comfrey root, dandelion root, burdock root, or ginseng may be utilized.

Vulnerary herbs promote healing of wounds, cuts, and broken bones. These herbs include calendula flowers, marshmallow root, comfrey root and leaf, and aloe vera. They are often added to formulas.

Blood tonics are prescribed for people with anemia and menstrual disorders, and after chronic disease and fatigue. Red clover, sassafras, yellow dock, and parsley are good tonics for the blood.

Everyone has individual organs that need constant attention and toning. This may result from diseased conditions or they may simply be congenitally weak areas in our bodies. The following list gives herbs for toning the various organs.

Organ	Herb For Toning
Heart	hawthorn berries
	motherwort
	borage
Liver	dandelion root
	Oregon grape root
	mandrake root
Gallbladder	wild yam
	Oregon grape root

Organ	Herb For Toning
Stomach	peppermint agrimony wormwood
Spleen	barberry bark parsley elecampane
Nerves	catnip skullcap hops lady's slipper valerian
Kidney	parsley prince's pine (pipsissewa) alfalfa
Colon	comfrey root and leaf slippery elm
Lungs	mullein coltsfoot comfrey leaf marshmallow root yerba santa
Pancreas	dandelion root Jerusalem artichokes string bean broth
Female Reproductive System	red raspberry leaf blessed thistle dong quai squawvine
Male Reproductive System	ginseng fo-ti blessed thistle vervain

THERAPEUTIC CONSTITUENTS OF HERBS

What makes some plants herbs or medicinal plants? Medicinal plants contain "active constituents" or chemicals that are recognized by the scientific community to have a known effect on humans and animals. All plants have some or all of these constituents in varying amounts.

Carbohydrates—These include sugars and starches.

Mucilage—These are slimy, gelatinous materials that are soothing to mucous membranes and skin. They are contained in agar, psyllium seeds, flax seeds, aloe vera, mullein, coltsfoot, slippery elm, marshmallow root, angelica root, and others.

Gums—These are sticky substances used for many cosmetic preparations because they are soothing and soft.

Glycosides—They are made of sugar and a non-sugar compound; they have very pronounced physiological effects on the physical body.

Cardiac glycosides—These have a powerful action on the heart muscle. Foxglove (from which we get the drug digitalis) contains digitoxin, digoxin, digitonin, and other glycosides; lily of the valley contains convallatoxin and others. Foxglove has toxic effects, so lily of the valley is preferred.

Anthraquinone glycosides—These have a laxative effect because they stimulate the smooth muscle in the large intestine. Cascara contains barbaloin and chrysaloin; aloe contains barbaloin; rhubarb bark contains emodin; senna contains emodin.

Thiocyanate glycosides—These have an irritating and emetic effect and are found principally in the mustard family. White mustard contains sinalbin; black mustard contains sinigrin.

Phenolic glycosides—These produce a disinfectant, astringent, and diuretic action. Uva ursi contains arbutin; iris contains iridin; chimaphila contains arbutin.

Flavonol glycosides—These are circulatory and cardiac stimulants; they are also anti-spasmodic and diuretic. Some, like rutin, hesperidin, and citrin, reduce the fragility of the capillaries and help the body to strengthen the circulatory system and lower blood pressure. These are found in buckwheat. Flavonoids are also essential to the absorption of Vitamin C.

Alcohol glycosides—The most important in this group is salicin, found in willow and poplar bark. It oxidizes to salicylic acid in the body, which is the constituent of aspirin.

Aldehyde glycosides—They include salinigrin, contained in willow bark, vanillin in vanilla beans, and amygdalin, which is contained in cherry bark, the pits of many fruits, and in bitter almonds.

Lactone glycosides—Coumarin and its derivatives are the most important. Coumarin is found in tonka beans, sweet vernal grass, sweet clover, and red clover. Coumarin derivatives of scopoletin are found in black haw and cramp bark.

Saponin glycosides—These form foaming solutions in water upon shaking. They are irritating to the mucous membranes and can destroy red blood cells. They have an expectorant effect on the body and can be destroyed by heat. Licorice root contains glycyrrhizin; wild yam contains botogenin and diosgenin; ginseng contains many of these glycosides.

Cyanophore glycosides—These yield hydrocyanic acid. Amygdalin or laetrile is in bitter almonds, the rose family, and sorghum.

Alkaloids—All alkaloids contain nitrogen. (Alkaloids end in -ine, but often have prefixes to denote alkaloid from the same source as quinine, quinidine, and hydroquinine.) Lobelia contains 14 alkaloids, lobeline being the strongest. Poison hemlock contains coniine, a powerful poison. Black pepper has alkaloids, as do all of the nightshade vegetables (eggplants, tomatoes, potatoes). Coffee contains caffeine, which is also in cocoa, tea, and kola. Periwinkle is endowed with vincristine, which is being used to treat Hodgkin's disease and other cancers. Coco leaves contain cocaine, used as a local anesthetic. Goldenseal has three alkaloids—hydrastine, berberine, and canadine. Hydrastine acts as an astringent to the mucous membranes. Oregon grape root contains berberine and ocycanthine; berberine also manifests as an astringent on the mucous membranes. Belladonna (nightshade family) contains atropine; it is used prior to surgery to inhibit secretions and relax muscles.

Tannins—All plant families are thought to contain tannins, which can be found in any part of the plant. They precipitate proteins and then combine with them to resist enzyme action. They protect abraded tissue while new tissue forms, and they are also antiseptic. They are useful for ulcers, diarrhea, bleeding (to constrict capillaries), burns, and wounds. Tannins are powerful astringents. Plants high in tannins include oak bark, rose leaves, uva ursi, peppermint, and sage. Tannins are water soluble but are destroyed by excessive heat and exposure to air.

Bitter Principles—These are not one chemical group but are of varied composition. The bitter principles have been shown to have valuable therapeutic effects. Through reflex action via the taste buds, they stimulate the secretion of all the digestive juices, thus stimulating the action of the liver, aiding hepatic elimination. Research is also being conducted on their antibiotic, anti-fungal, and anti-tumor actions. Bitters can act as nervines as well. Some bitters are hops, gentian, dandelion, chicory, nux vomica, and buckbean.

Volatile Oils—This is the part that gives plants their odors. They are called volatile because they turn from a liquid to a gas quickly. Volatile oils are found in the glandular structure of one or more plant parts; they may attract polli-nating insects to the plant. The various actions of volatile oils are:

Antiseptic—thyme, mints, pepper

Antibacterial—garlic, onions

Anthelmintic (expels worms from the digestive tract)—wormwood, worm-seed, fennel

Anti-inflammatory—wintergreen, lavender, willow, poplar

Carminative (stimulates peristalsis and relaxes the stomach)—anise, caraway, spearmint, peppermint

Diuretic (increases elimination of urine)—juniper berries

Febrifuge (reduces fevers)—yarrow, chamomile, elder flowers, peppermint

Irritant (to increase circulation)—cayenne, eucalyptus, cinnamon, rosemary, tansy

Insect repellent—citronella, pennyroyal, peppermint

Resins and Balsams—Resins are hard, transparent, meltable substances, insoluble in water, and of a complex chemical nature. They are used in var-nishes, inks, and sealing wax. Balsams are resinous mixtures containing ben-zoic acid. Benzoin is used as an expectorant, a stimulant, and a diuretic.

Steroids—Steroids are compounds widely distributed in plants: cholesterol in ferns, fungi, algae; hormones in wild yam, black cohosh.

HERBAL PREPARATIONS

Teas

Herbs for medicinal use may be taken in various forms. The most common form is a tea. Teas include infusions and decoctions. In an *infusion*, 1 ounce of dried herb is steeped in 1 pint (2 cups) boiling water for about 10 minutes (1 t. herb to 1 cup water). It can be steeped in a teapot, or the herb can be put in a tea ball. Leaves, stems, flowers, and berries are infused. Roots and barks are decocted. In a *decoction*, the herbs are simmered in water 15–20 minutes. About 1 t. herb to 1 cup of water is used, but extra water should be added since some of it evaporates.

Tinctures

A very common method of using herbs is in the form of tinctures. People often find tinctures more convenient to use than teas, though there is some objection to the idea that alcohol is necessary in making a tincture. Some people feel that the alcohol can be removed by placing the tincture in heated water; alcohol boils at a lower temperature than water. The tincture still has the vibration of alcohol and affects the blood sugar.

Gelatin Capsules and Pills

When the herb has a bad taste, one often pulverizes it and puts the powdered form in gelatin capsules. This is done with goldenseal powder. The disadvantage of using gelatin capsules is that they are difficult to assimilate. Vegetarians also do not like using them. Pills are more acceptable to many. Herbs do not have to be so finely powdered for pills. A small amount of slippery elm or other mucilaginous herb powder is used and mixed with water until a doughy consistency is reached. Gum arabic dissolved in water is also a good adhesive. The pills can then be dried in the oven at low heat or in the warm air.

Smoking

For relief of respiratory conditions and bronchial infections, certain herbs are smoked. A small amount of herb is smoked in a pipe or water pipe. The lungs are filled with smoke, and then it's exhaled. For a single treatment, the smoke should be inhaled 6–10 times. Herbs used for this purpose are mullein, lobelia, yerba santa, and coltsfoot.

Syrups

Syrups are used for coughs and sore throats. Two ounces of herb are used per quart of water, and this is boiled down to 1 pint. After it is strained, honey or glycerine is used. Syrups may be given in doses of 1 to 2 teaspoons daily for several days. Herbs commonly made into syrups include wild cherry bark, licorice root, comfrey root, and small amounts of lobelia for calming.

Salves

Salves are ointments that are applied to the skin which can be used for burns, cuts, external injuries, and wounds. The best way to make a salve is to extract the herbs in hot oil, starting with roots and barks (about 2 hours), adding leaves and flowers (1 more hour). Afterwards, melted wax is added, and a small amount of gum benzoin or tincture of benzoin for preservation. Herbs used in salves are comfrey leaves, plantain, chickweed, St. John's wort, goldenseal, and myrrh.

Liniments

Liniments are herbal extracts rubbed into the skin for treating strained muscles and ligaments and for inflammatory conditions such as arthritis. Four ounces of dried herbs are placed in a bottle with 1 pint of vinegar, alcohol, or massage oil, and this is allowed to extract for 3 days. Liniments usually include stimulant herbs, such as cayenne, and oils of aromatic herbs, such as eucalyptus and wintergreen.

Poultices and Plasters

A poultice is a warm, moist application of powdered or macerated herbs that is applied to the skin to relieve inflammation and to promote the cleansing of the affected area. Poultices can draw out infections as well as toxins and foreign bodies. Herbs used include comfrey, plantain, and marshmallow root. To relieve pain and muscle spasm, herbs such as lobelia, catnip, vervain, and valerian can be used.

In a plaster, the herbal materials are placed between two thin pieces of linen or are combined in a thick material and applied to the skin. An example would be a mustard plaster.

Fomentations or Compresses

A fomentation or compress is used to treat swellings, pain, cold, and flu. It can stimulate the circulation of the blood or lymph in the area of the body to which it is applied. Sometimes herbs that are too strong to be used internally can be used externally with the body absorbing only a small amount.

A compress is prepared by making an herbal tea and dipping a towel or cloth into the tea. Then apply it, as hot as possible, to the affected area. The towel can be covered with a dry flannel cloth or heating pad.

Ginger compresses are helpful in stimulating circulation in certain areas and reducing inflammation. Grate fresh ginger root and put in cheesecloth or a tea ball. Make a strong ginger root tea, and then dip a towel or cloth into this mixture and apply to the affected area. Ginger compresses on the colon are helpful in cases of constipation or blockage.

Bolus

A *bolus* is a suppository which is made by adding powdered herbs to cocoa butter until the mixture forms a firm consistency. It is then placed in the refrigerator to harden, and should be warmed to room temperature before use. The bolus is rolled into strips about 3/4" thick and cut into segments 1" long. It is inserted into the rectum to treat cysts and into the vagina for infections. Herbs used in boluses include antibiotics, such as garlic, goldenseal, or chaparral, and demulcents, such as comfrey root and slippery elm.

HARVESTING HERBS

In order for herbal medicines to be the most effective, herbs should be of high quality. The quality depends on where they are grown, when they are harvested, how they are dried and preserved, how they are stored, and the duration of storage.

Dried herbs bought in stores are generally a couple of years old unless they are harvested locally and brought right to the store. Many of them are imported from other countries and different areas of the United States. To obtain herbs as fresh as possible, individuals should harvest their own herbs (at least those that are available in the area). The time to harvest herbs is when they contain the highest amount of active constituents. This varies from place to place, depending on the growing season, the amount of sunlight, and other factors.

Leaves are picked just before the plant is about to flower. At this time, the energy is focused in the upper portion of the plant. The best time of day to pick herbs is after the morning dew has dried, but before the hot Sun has caused the essential oils to evaporate. Flowers are picked before reaching full bloom. Berries and fruits may be obtained at peak ripeness when they are about to fall from the plant; this occurs usually in late summer.

Barks and twigs of trees are collected in the spring when the sap rises and the leaves first appear. Roots are gathered in the fall when the sap returns to the ground and the berries or seeds are mature.

Several guidelines are important when collecting wild plants:

1. Don't harvest plants that are protected, endangered, or a rare species.
2. Be sure in your identification of the plant. Field guides with colored photographs are helpful. If unsure, check with a local botanist. (For example, the parsley-carrot family has edible and poisonous members which are difficult to tell apart.)
3. Look for the "grandmother" plant (the largest one). Ask permission of that plant to harvest some of the surrounding plants. Tell the plants what you are picking them for. Don't pick tender, young plants. Only pick one out of five plants in an area so that they can repopulate.
4. Disturb the area as little as possible when picking. Cover any holes, and do not walk on plants.
5. Have clippers, scissors, or other cutting tools for leaves and stems. Do not pick plants up by the roots unless you are going to use the whole root.
6. Collect plants that are far removed from roadsides where there may be automobile exhaust. Be aware of areas that may be chemically sprayed.
7. Dry plants immediately upon returning home.

DRYING AND PRESERVING HERBS

Plant tops should be washed, allowed to dry, and then hung in a well-ventilated, shaded area. The plant may be tied in bundles and hung upside down so that the sap runs from the stems into the leaves. They may also be spread out on a screen and turned each day. Roots and barks are scrubbed and chopped before drying. The pieces should not be more than an inch thick. They also may be dried on a screen and turned daily. Depending on how warm the area is where the herbs are drying, it takes from three to five days.

It is important to store herbs well since medicinal properties are destroyed by heat, bright light, exposure to air, bacteria, and fungi. They should be kept in a cool, dry place with minimum exposure to air and sunlight. After a few days, they should be checked to be sure there is no mold or moisture in the jar.

Herbs should also be labeled with their name and date collected. After a year, they should be checked and restocked. When they begin to lose their color and smell, they may be set aside for herbal baths. Herbs with aromatic oils lose potency first; barks, roots, and seeds maintain potency for a longer period.

Oils may last in the refrigerator or another cool place for several years. Salves and lotions may be preserved by adding a small amount of tincture of benzoin.

HERBAL MATERIA MEDICA

The rest of this chapter discusses the uses of particular herbs, and is organized by their function.

Alteratives—These are also known as "blood cleansers"; they cleanse the blood and the lymph and restore the body to its proper functioning.

Echinacea—It is an antiseptic, antibiotic, and anti-toxic. Echinacea is a prime remedy against bacterial and viral attacks; it helps the body rid itself of microbial infections. It is used for infections of the respiratory tract, such as laryngitis and tonsillitis, and catarrhal conditions of the nose and sinuses. It's also beneficial for eczema from blood conditions as well as gastric and duodenal ulcers. As a decoction, it may be used for pyorrhea and gingivitis.

Yellow dock—This is used for chronic skin complaints like psoriasis. Yellow dock is also a mild laxative since it increases bile flow; its action on the gall-bladder makes it a helpful herb in treating jaundice. It is high in iron and thus used to treat anemia. It combines well with dandelion, burdock, and cleavers. As a salve, it is good for skin diseases and swelling.

Burdock root—This root is excellent for skin conditions which result from dry and scaly skin, including eczema and psoriasis. Through its bitter principle, it stimulates digestive juices and bile secretion. It is used in the treatment of arthritis, rheumatism, lumbago, and sciatica. It is also used to help the kidneys function and works through the kidneys to help clear the blood of harmful acids. Burdock seeds made into an extraction are good for skin and kidney diseases. Burdock can also be utilized as a fomentation for wounds, swellings, and hemorrhoids.

Sarsaparilla root—This is used in treating skin problems and is frequently combined with sassafras, yellow dock, and cleavers. Sarsaparilla root is also used to treat rheumatism, arthritis, and gout. It contains hormone-like substances and thus is valuable in formulas for glandular balancing to alleviate discomforts associated with menopause and irregular menstruation.

Anti-spasmodics—These ease spasms or cramps in various parts of the body.

Cramp bark—Cramp bark is helpful in relieving muscle cramps, spasms, and also in uterine muscle problems. Thus, it is a good herb for painful cramps associated with menstruation or possible miscarriage. For uterine cramps, it is often used with black haw and valerian.

Lady's slipper—A widely used nervine and anti-spasmodic, lady's slipper is used for states of anxiety as well as pains in the nerves. It is a good tonic for exhausted nervous systems because it improves circulation and nutrition to the nerves.

Lobelia—Lobelia is one of the strongest relaxants for the central and autonomic nervous systems. It is often used in combination with other herbs to increase their effectiveness. Its particular use is in bronchial asthma where it is often combined with ephedra, cayenne, and grindelia.

Astringents—These contract tissue and can thus reduce secretions and discharges. Astringents contain tannins.

Eyebright—Eyebright is excellent for problems of mucous membranes. It is used for eye problems in inflammatory conditions as well as for stinging and weeping eyes. It is drunk as a tea and also used in compresses. It is an anticatarrhal and may be used for nasal catarrh and sinusitis in combination with goldenseal, goldenrod, or elder flowers. Eyebright also aids the liver in cleansing the blood.

Barberry—Barberry is a bitter tonic with mild laxative effects. It promotes the flow of bile and is indicated where there is inflammation of the gallbladder and where the liver is congested as it is in the case of jaundice. It is also able to reduce an enlarged spleen.

Goldenseal—One of the most useful of the medicinal plants, goldenseal is a powerful toner to the mucous membranes. Goldenseal leaf is excellent for ulcers, colitis, and gastritis as well as catarrhal conditions of the upper respiratory tract. The leaf is infused. Externally, as a paste, it may be applied to eczema, poison ivy or oak, acne, ringworm, and other skin infections. Internally, it may be drunk as a tea or taken powdered in capsules.

Carminatives—Carminatives stimulate peristalsis in the digestive system and relaxation in the stomach. In doing this, they help to expel gas.

Aniseed—Aniseed is good for flatulence and intestinal colic. It is usually ground up and mixed with ground fennel seeds, caraway seeds, and dill seeds. Aniseed also works as an expectorant and anti-spasmodic. It is helpful for bronchitis and where there is coughing as in whooping cough. In these conditions, it is often mixed with coltsfoot, white horehound, and lobelia.

Caraway—Caraway is used for flatulence and intestinal colic; it stimulates the appetite and helps in the treatment of diarrhea. It is often used in combination with aniseed, fennel seed, and dill seed (ground up and made into a tea). Caraway is also used as an anti-spasmodic in bronchitis and bronchial asthma.

Dill—Dill is another herb used for flatulence and intestinal colic, especially in children; it is combined with the two herbs listed above and with fennel. In addition, ground dill seeds stimulate the flow of milk in nursing mothers, as does caraway.

Fennel—This is excellent as a stomach and intestinal remedy to relieve flatulence while also stimulating the appetite and digestion. It has a similarity to aniseed in its calming action on bronchitis and coughs. It is also used to flavor cough remedies and increase the flow of milk in nursing mothers (ground up and made into a tea).

Peppermint—Peppermint is one of the best carminatives; it stimulates bile and digestive juices, thereby aiding conditions of flatulence, dyspepsia, and intestinal colic; it also helps ulcerative colitis and Crohn's disease. It allays feelings of nausea, especially during pregnancy, and is valuable in the treatment of fevers in colds and flus.

Demulcents—These contain mucilage and are soothing to irritated or inflamed internal tissue.

Comfrey—Comfrey root and leaf is one of the most useful and versatile herbs. The presence of *allantoin* helps wounds to heal internally and externally. Comfrey is an excellent healing agent in gastric and duodenal ulcers and in ulcerative colitis and hiatal hernia. For these conditions, it is often combined with marshmallow root and meadowsweet. It is also used for coughs and bronchitis where it soothes and reduces irritation; in these cases it is often combined with coltsfoot, elecampane, and white horehound. Comfrey is used externally in salves for skin irritations and as a poultice.

Irish moss—This has a high amount of mucilage and is used for both gastritis and ulcers as a tea (the dried herb is infused). It is also used in the food industry to make jellies and aspic. Its main use, however, is for respiratory problems like bronchitis.

Marshmallow—Marshmallow root and leaf have a high mucilage content. The root is used for digestive problems and on the skin, while the leaf is used more for the lungs and urinary system. For inflammations of the digestive tract like gastritis, peptic ulcers, and colitis, the root is used in combination with comfrey and sometimes slippery elm. For bronchitis and coughs, the leaf is often used with comfrey, licorice root, and white horehound.

Slippery elm—The bark of slippery elm is soothing and nutritive for inflamed mucous membranes in colitis, ulcers, and gastritis. The powdered bark is used as a nutritive food and may be mixed in juices and cereals. Externally, slippery elm is used as a poultice for boils and abscesses.

Aloe—The juice from the leaves of the aloe vera plant is helpful in digestive complaints since it soothes the lining of the intestine. It is also helpful for flatulence and constipation; drinking 1/4 or 1/3 cup of this juice will aid elimination. Externally, aloe gel is excellent for burns, sunburn, and insect bites.

Diaphoretics—These promote sweating and aid the skin in the elimination of toxins.

Cayenne—Cayenne is one of the most versatile of the stimulating herbs. The powder can be used in soups, salads, or in cooking; or it can be infused and drunk with water. In the circulatory system, it regulates blood flow and strengthens the heart and arteries. In the digestive system, it is used for flatulence, dyspepsia, and colic. It is also a good source of Vitamin P, one of the bioflavonoids which helps to assimilate Vitamin C.

Elder—Elder has many uses; the bark, flowers, berries, and leaves are utilized. The leaves, flowers, and berries are used for treatment of colds and flu as well as for the inflammation of the upper respiratory tract like sinusitis. Elder is also a good diuretic. It may be combined with peppermint, yarrow, or hyssop for colds and flus, and with goldenrod for nasal catarrh.

Garlic—Garlic is the most universally used of the medicinal herbs. It is effective against bacteria, parasites, and viruses. It aids the immune system and is often used in combination with echinacea. In the digestive tract, it supports natural flora while killing pathogenic bacteria. It helps circulation and is used for colds and flus. Garlic can be eaten as cloves, cooked with food, or taken in capsules of garlic oil.

Ginger—Ginger is used in feverish conditions to promote perspiration. It is also used to stimulate circulation in cases of chilblains or cramps. As a carminative, it promotes gastric secretions and is used for dyspepsia, flatulence, and colic. It is also helpful for motion sickness. Ginger root is simmered, often with other herbs, and used as a tea.

Diuretics—These increase the secretion and elimination of urine.

Corn silk—Corn silk consists of the fine soft threads from the flowering corn; it is best used fresh but may be dried first. It is helpful in irritations of the urinary system. Combined with other herbs like couchgrass, bearberry, or yarrow, it treats cystitis, urethritis, and prostatitis.

Cleavers—Cleavers is one of the finest diuretics. It is used for all kidney and bladder problems, particularly for stones and gravel. It is also an excellent alterative as well as a toner for the lymphatic system (used for swollen glands, tonsillitis, and adenoid problems). Cleavers is beneficial for skin conditions when it is combined with yellow dock and burdock and applied often.

Dandelion—Dandelion root and its leaves are used. It is an excellent diuretic because it is a natural source of potassium; therefore, it stimulates kidney function without the loss of potassium. Dandelion root is also used as a *cholagogue* in inflammation and congestion of the liver and gallbladder. It is the best tonic for the liver and may be used with barberry or balmony.

Gravel root—Gravel root is used primarily for kidney stones or gravel. It may be used in urinary infections like cystitis and urethritis as well as in the treatment of rheumatism or gout. It is often used with parsley or hydrangea for kidney stones or gravel.

Juniper berries—Juniper berries are an excellent antiseptic in conditions such as cystitis. They should be avoided in kidney disease as they are stimulating to the kidney nephrons. They may also be used in conditions of rheumatism or arthritis.

Nettles—Nettle leaves are one of the most useful herbs available. They are high in iron, potassium, silicon, and Vitamin C. Nettles are used for anemia, as a "blood purifier," and for nosebleeds and other hemorrhages in the body.

The tea is also an expectorant for the lungs in combination with comfrey, mullein, and white horehound.

Parsley—Parsley has many usages; primarily, it is a diuretic, an *emmenagogue*, stimulating the menstrual cycle, and a *carminative* to ease flatulence. Parsley is a good source of Vitamin C, potassium, and other nutrients.

Nervines—These tone and strengthen the nervous system. Some act as relaxants; some act as stimulants.

Chamomile—One of the most widely used herbs, chamomile is calming for restlessness, anxiety, nervous stomach, and insomnia. It is especially good for children who suffer from digestive upsets. It eases flatulence and dyspeptic pain and is also helpful in cases of gastritis. As an inhalant over a steam bath, it helps nasal catarrh.

Hops—Hops have a strong effect on the central nervous system and are, therefore, used in the treatment of insomnia, often combined with valerian and passion flower. Hops also have an effect on the liver and gallbladder and increase the flow of bile.

Passion flower—Passion flower treats insomnia and is also used as an antispasmodic in Parkinson's disease and seizures. It is effective in neuralgia and in shingles (infection of nerves).

Scullcap—Scullcap is one of the most widely used nervines. It is used in the treatment of nervous tension, seizures, epilepsy, and hysteria. It has the quality of renewing the entire nervous system.

St. John's wort—St. John's wort is a very versatile plant. It has a sedative effect internally and thus is used for anxiety, restlessness, and irritability (particularly the irritability that often accompanies menopause). Externally, it is an anti-inflammatory for use in healing wounds and bruises, mild burns, and varicose veins.

Valerian—Valerian is one of the most effective relaxing nervines and is often used in orthodox medicine. It relieves tension and anxiety, is used for insomnia (often with hops and passion flower), and has an anti-spasmodic effect that is helpful in relieving cramps (including menstrual cramps) and intestinal colic.

Vervain—This herb is helpful in cases of depression and melancholy and is often mixed with scullcap, oats, and lady's slipper for this. It is also used for seizures and hysteria in addition to acting as a *diaphoretic* in the early stages of fever.

Stimulants—These quicken the physiological functions of the body.

Cayenne—see *Diaphoretics*

Ginger—see *Diaphoretics*

Mustard—Internally, mustard is used as a stimulant for colds, fevers, and flus. The mustard flower is infused as a tea and drunk. Externally, mustard stimulates the circulation to a particular area of the body, which relieves muscular and skeletal pain. A poultice of mustard will also help bronchitis.

Toners—These tone various organs or the whole body. There are specific tonic herbs for various body systems.

Circulatory System

Hawthorn berries—Hawthorn berries tone the heart and circulatory system, either stimulating or depressing the heart, depending on its need. They may be used for heart palpitations and also for treatment of high blood pressure, arteriosclerosis, and recurrent chest pains.

Motherwort—Motherwort is a good tonic to strengthen the heart; it is used for rapid heartbeat as well as conditions associated with anxiety and tension. This herb is also useful in certain menstrual conditions, such as delayed menstruation, and is a good tonic for menopausal changes.

Digestive System

Comfrey root—see *Demulcents*

Marshmallow root—see *Demulcents*

Slippery elm—see *Demulcents*

Agrimony—Agrimony's combination of bitter and astringent properties make it a good toner for the digestive system since it can stimulate liver and digestive secretions. In cases of mucous colitis, diarrhea, and appendicitis, agrimony works well.

Dandelion root—see *Diuretics*

Nervous System

Chamomile—see *Nervines*

Vervain—see *Nervines*

Lady's slipper—see *Anti-spasmodics*

Scullcap—see *Nervines*

Respiratory System

Coltsfoot—Coltsfoot is soothing to the mucous linings and has an expectorant and anti-spasmodic action as well. This makes it helpful in respiratory conditions, bronchitis, asthma, and whooping cough. For coughs, it is often used with white horehound and mullein.

Comfrey root and leaves—see *Demulcents*

Elecampane—Elecampane has an expectorant action, soothes the mucous linings by relaxing them, and is antibacterial. It may be used where there is catarrh formed as in bronchitis and emphysema. Its bitter quality also helps to stimulate digestion. It is often used in combination with coltsfoot, yarrow, and white horehound.

Reproductive System

Black cohosh—Black cohosh is an excellent herb for toning the female reproductive system. It balances the sex hormones and is used in cases of delayed menstruation, painful menstruation, and menopausal conditions. It is also a relaxing nervine utilized in the treatment of rheumatic as well as muscular and neurological pains.

Ginseng—Ginseng root comes from the Orient; it is a toner for the male hormonal system and generally raises the vitality. It helps normalize blood pressure and reduces blood cholesterol. It also reduces blood sugar levels and is thus helpful in diabetes.

Dong quai—Dong quai is an herb from China that aids the female reproductive system. It is helpful for menstrual cramps, irregular menstruation, and menopause. It is also a good "blood purifier" and is used in treating anemia as well as circulatory problems.

Raspberry—These leaves create a wonderful tea for the female organs. Used throughout pregnancy, it eases cramps and pain in childbirth. It is also used for menstrual cramps and normalizing the menstrual cycle. Raspberry leaf is combined with other herbs like uva ursi and squawvine to treat vaginal discharge.

Squawvine—Squawvine was used by Native American women during pregnancy to assure proper development of the child and to help promote proper lactation. It is excellent for painful and irregular menstruation, relieving congestion in the ovaries and uterus. It is often combined with raspberry leaf. If the berries are crushed and added to a tincture of myrrh for a few days, it will provide a good fomentation for sore nipples.

Urinary System

Gravel—see *Diuretics*

Nettles—see *Diuretics*

Parsley—see *Diuretics*

CHAPTER 11:
BODYWORK THERAPIES

In order to keep our bodies free of toxins and in physical alignment, it is helpful to have regular bodywork. Bodywork is different from exercise; when we have various types of bodywork, our bodies are shaped and re-aligned, tensions in muscles are removed, and energy is brought in through the unblocking of certain meridians. Bodywork therapies help us to balance our physical vehicles and make us aware of our body's complexity. Within our bodies, we contain the four elements. Earth is seen in the structure of our body, our bones and joints, the way our body is held together. Techniques such as osteopathy and chiropractic help us with our Earth element by helping us understand how our bodies have been put together. Water, our emotional body, may be balanced through sensual massage techniques such as Swedish massage and Lomi-lomi. We can also get in touch with our deepest feelings and release old modes of behavior through techniques that involve deep tissue work such as Rolfing, Bioenergetics, and Reichian work. Fire, magnetism, is transmitted through therapies that transmit electromagnetic energy such as Acupressure, Shiatsu, Jin Shin, and Polarity therapy. Air, the breath of life, is transmitted through all of these techniques and especially through those that work with the subtle body such as Therapeutic touch, Reiki, and hands on healing.

The most important requirement in choosing a particular bodywork therapy is the alchemy between the healer and the one being healed. Through this alchemy the vital force (*prana, chi*) is transmitted. It is also helpful to work with healers who are familiar with several different therapies so that they can be used in combination.

Bodywork therapies may be divided into several different categories:

1. Those that work with the body structure such as osteopathy and chiropractic.

2. Sensual and relaxing types of massage like Swedish massage and Lomi-lomi.
3. Massage techniques based on deep tissue work which break down body armor and release pent-up emotions. Such techniques include Rolfing, Bioenergetics, and Reichian work.
4. Therapies that work with the electromagnetic currents in the body such as acupuncture, acupressure, Shiatsu, Jin Shin, polarity therapy, and reflexology (see Chapter 2).
5. Healing techniques that work with the subtle or etheric body (see Chapter 2).

BODY STRUCTURE TECHNIQUES

Osteopathy

Osteopathy, the first structural or manipulative therapy, was developed by Dr. Andrew Still, a physician from Missouri; the first college of osteopathy was established in Missouri in 1897. The basis of osteopathy is that when spinal problems exist, biochemical changes occur which interfere with normal nerve transmission and circulation. This affects not only the muscles and skeleton, but also the circulation and all the organs of the body.

Interdependence between structure and function is the basis of osteopathic work; if the musculoskeletal structure of the body is abnormal in any way, then the function also becomes altered. Optimum function depends on unimpeded flow of blood and nerve impulses. Mechanical manipulation can be helpful in correcting the musculoskeletal abnormalities and allowing more *chi* to enter the body. Some osteopaths also work with nutrition, preventive medicine, and fitness in achieving balance; but most osteopaths usually have time only for the manipulations. I have found osteopathic manipulations very helpful in releasing blocked energy and increasing the vital flow.

Chiropractic

Chiropractic work is based on the theory that when the vertebrae of the spine are not in alignment, an unlimited amount of symptoms can occur. *Chiropractic* was developed by Dr. David Palmer in Iowa and practiced in the United States as early as 1895. Palmer believed that misaligned spinal segments interfere with the passage of vital forces or nerve impulses. Manual adjustments of parts of the spine promote the health of the tissues supplied by the appropriate nerves.

The spine needs to be kept moving or aligned for the vital energy to flow. Chiropractic works with the 31 pairs of spinal nerves that travel with an artery and a vein. The nervous system is the communicator that uses electrical energy to send impulses to the blood. Blockages in the spine affect our entire being since blood carries nutrients to the body. Each vertebrae in the body is connected to a certain organ; when this vertebrae is out of alignment, various symptoms may occur such as headaches, sinus trouble, earaches, and pain around the eyes.

Chiropractors adjust the spine in many different ways. Some make strong forceful adjustments while others work more subtly. A school of chiropractors known as Network Chiropractic uses very subtle movements on the spine that are designed to balance the nervous system.

Of all the alternative body therapies, chiropractic is the one most recognized by the medical establishment. There are many chiropractic colleges and most health insurance plans include chiropractic work.

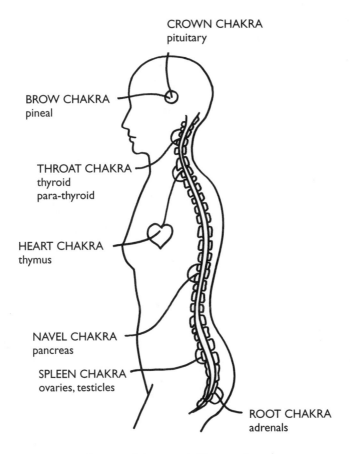

CROWN CHAKRA
pituitary

BROW CHAKRA
pineal

THROAT CHAKRA
thyroid
para-thyroid

HEART CHAKRA
thymus

NAVEL CHAKRA
pancreas

SPLEEN CHAKRA
ovaries, testicles

ROOT CHAKRA
adrenals

Diagram of Autonomic Nervous System

Craniosacral Therapy

Craniosacral therapy manipulates the skull bones so that they move in sync with one another, allowing the cerebro-spinal fluid to circulate freely. During the manipulation process, practitioners of craniosacral therapy remove the stresses that have accumulated in the membranes that support the brain and spinal column.

All of the bruises and blows to our head that we have ever received—including the birth process—have probably pushed the skull bones out of alignment so that they move improperly. This interferes with the quality of our energy and often gives us headaches and other problems related to the temporo mandibular joint (TMJ).

A craniosacral therapist holds the skull gently and attunes to the rhythm of the individual patient. With gentle movements, the therapist re-balances the fluid and/or balances the bones. The treatment often causes the patient to drift off into a state of deep consciousness.

Two pioneers in this area of work have been Dr. William Sutherland and Dr. John Upledger. Dr. Sutherland experimented by wrapping his head with bandages so that his skull bones could not move. In doing this, he found an immediate change in his respiration. He felt that the cranial respiratory system was the primary one, with the skull designed to expand and contract. Sutherland concluded that restrictions in the craniosacral rhythm may be implicated in conditions such as migraines and depression.

Dr. John Upledger also participated in these investigations at Michigan State University's College of Osteopathic Medicine. He teaches craniosacral therapy to many students at his institute in Florida. Craniosacral work has proven effective in relieving migraine headaches, ringing in the ears, cerebral palsy, and TMJ-related joint pain. Many problems in other parts of the body have also been helped by this therapy.

Ortho-bionomy

Ortho-bionomy is a noninvasive osteopathically based form of body therapy which is highly effective in working with injuries and pain that involve postural and structural imbalances. Ortho-bionomy helps to alleviate acute and chronic pain by reducing muscle tension, soothing the joints, increasing flexibility, improving circulation, and relaxing the entire body. The term "Ortho-bionomy" comes from *ortho*, meaning correct or straight, *bio*, which is "life," and *nomy*, "the study of."

Ortho-bionomy was developed by Dr. Arthur Lincoln Pauls, a British osteopath, who searched for a way to work with the body that honored the body's inherent wisdom. From his experience as a Judo instructor and through his training as an osteopath, he found ways of working with the body which consisted of exaggerating the body's postures, thereby permitting the body's self-healing process to create greater balance and alignment. He discovered that by working *with* the body and not against it, the body could find balance on its own without the use of force. Dr. Pauls began teaching this work in the United States in 1976 as well as throughout Europe.

An Ortho-bionomy session can be done clothed or bare-skinned if therapeutic massage is incorporated, which it usually is. The practitioner locates a tension point in the body and then begins moving the body into a pain release position for that joint, releasing the "locked" muscles that are causing sensitivity. With one hand on the tension point, the practitioner rotates a limb to find a pain-relieving position and cradles the body in this position. Holding the position for a few minutes, the body is rocked slightly. The rocking motion enhances integration—the correction of the relationship between all muscles at the joint. After returning the body to its fully extended position and pressing the tension point again, sensitivity decreases.

The key to Ortho-bionomy is loosening tightened muscles around troubled joints. This enables the relaxed muscle to return to its normal shape and function. Ortho-bionomy is a cooperative effort between the client and practitioner; both are working together to release the tensions. Outside of the sessions, the client becomes aware of attitudes, emotions, and movements that are creating bodily tensions. This helps to maintain the relaxation of the muscles and freedom of movement. My own experience with Ortho-bionomy has been very positive; with the alleviation of the tension in the muscles, my body feels much looser and the *chi* is able to circulate more freely.

SENSUAL AND RELAXING MASSAGE TECHNIQUES

Swedish Massage

When most people talk about massage, they generally mean Swedish massage. In the early part of the 20th century, Peter Long of Sweden developed a system of massage strokes that integrates ancient Oriental techniques with more modern principles of anatomy and physiology. The system was then introduced into the United States by Dr. S. W. Mitchell.

Swedish massage emphasizes several basic strokes applied to the soft tissue of the body, often quite vigorously. There are many benefits to this type of massage. It helps improve circulation by encouraging the movement of blood through the veins, toward the heart. It aids in balancing the musculature, relieving tensions in the body, and soreness in the shoulders, neck, and back. Massage also has a tranquilizing effect on the central nervous system. It enables people to become aware of where tensions exist in the body and how to prevent them.

Among the conditions that massage benefits are arthritis, bronchial asthma, indigestion and constipation, neuromuscular disorders such as multiple sclerosis, spastic paralysis, and flaccid paralysis, edema and swelling of the limbs, and back, neck, and shoulder pain. Massage helps in circulation to the heart and also digestive organs, in relieving pain by working on the muscles attached to the sore spots, and in clearing out phlegm and mucus in bronchial tubes. Most important, massage helps to release stress and tension in the body as well as emotional blocks that have accumulated.

Lomi-lomi

Lomi-lomi is a type of massage practiced by the Hawaiian Kahunas. (*Kahuna* means "keeper of the secret.") Lomi-lomi is a combination of Swedish massage with baths, chiropractic, osteopathy, and the ancient practice of "laying on of hands." Lomi-lomi practitioners use their elbows and forearms as well as their hands; their strokes are vigorous and they incorporate the technique of massaging away from the heart (as in the Orient and South America) and move energy toward the extremities. It takes a special kind of spiritual energy to practice the real Lomi-lomi; though today, many simply use the physical massage techniques.

DEEP TISSUE WORK

Rolfing

Rolfing, also known as structural integration, was developed by Dr. Ida Rolf in the 1930s; it is a technique which encourages the freeing of the body, mind, and emotions from their conditioning. Dr. Rolf believes that muscular imbalance in the body can be a shield or armoring which protects a person from deep hurts that have occurred throughout life. These armorings pull on the body, causing a limitation of movement and rigidity. The body's rigid patterns reflect mental and emotional attitudes.

Another important concept in rolfing is that of gravity. Distortion of the body is accentuated by gravity. Rolfing involves the loosening and lengthening of specific muscles and the fascia (the envelope of connective tissue which houses muscles, tendons, ligaments, and nerves). Misalignments, which may have been distorted by previous accidents or illness, by fear and other conditioning, resume their normal functions.

A rolfing treatment usually involves 10 sessions. Specific sessions focus on various parts of the body. As old muscle patterns are broken up, the individual may experience emotions and attitudes from childhood which have been restrictive.

Rolfing sessions are not necessarily painful, although the work is deep. Rolfing can vary from one practitioner to another; my own experience with two different rolfers taught me that the particular practitioner can make the sessions very different and gear them to the individual. Many people have changed their posture as well as attitudes after being rolfed.

Aston Patterning

Aston patterning combines bodywork with movement. Judith Aston began studying with Ida Rolf in doing deep tissue work. Then she added her own ideas concerning the asymmetrical movement of the body. Aston felt that people move like spirals in space, not straight, and that each person has a unique pattern of movement.

In Aston patterning, the practitioner looks for areas of tension in the body and maps these on a body chart. Then, the person stands and moves; a videotape is made to show the type of movement that is unique to the individual. Along with working on moving, bodywork is given that involves connective-tissue massage with gentle strokes that move the tissue in an asymmetrical spiral. Work with the breath is also incorporated to promote flexible and graceful movements.

Reichian Therapy and Bioenergetics (See Chapter 4.)

CHAPTER 12:
EXERCISE

I n our Western society, one of the most harmful habits to fall into is that of
not moving. Many of us have jobs that keep us rooted to one spot, and
when we return home, we often choose sedentary activities such as watching
television or reading a book. We may have chores that require plenty of movement but we do them in a state of annoyance or exhaustion, which further
stresses our bodies.

Physical exercise is a necessity in maintaining the health of the body and
spirit. Exercise affects metabolism, digestion, circulation, stamina, and emotional balance. Remaining sedentary for extensive time periods leads to a sluggish metabolism, poor digestion, impaired circulation, moodiness, and
depression. Exercise helps the body to burn off toxins as well as assimilate
important minerals such as calcium, magnesium, and iron.

One of the primary functions of exercise is to stretch and reshape the
body. There are several types of exercise that stretch the body—Hatha yoga,
gymnastics, dance, as well as Feldenkrais and Alexander work (Feldenkrais
and Alexander work include both bodywork and exercise), which also help to
reshape the body. Another function of exercise is to increase vital force. Tai
Chi, Chi Gung, and the various forms of yoga strengthen the vital force
through focusing and working with the breath. Aerobic-type exercise (which
includes running, jogging, aerobic dance, and aerobic walking) increases the
heart rate and circulation.

Exercise is also a way of interrelating with nature; hiking, swimming,
canoeing, sailing, and skiing enable one to connect with the forces of nature
and become invigorated through this interchange.

Opening up to higher states of awareness is another function of exercise.
Physical disciplines such as Tai Chi, Chi Gung, and the various forms of yoga

work with the body and breath in ways that produce a calm and meditative state. The martial arts—Aikido, Karate, and Judo—utilize psychological and spiritual wisdom in their practice.

There are many forms of exercise available. Individual and team sports like tennis, basketball, racquetball, soccer, and swimming have been popular throughout the years. Many of our ancient cultures such as those of the Greeks, Romans, and Mayans held games which were not simply vehicles for exercise but a means to re-enact certain deep truths and wisdom. The Sioux also had a game (called Tapa Wanka Yap, the "throwing of the ball") in which the presence of the Great Spirit was revealed to the players. China, Japan, and Korea developed the martial arts which focus on mastering higher states of consciousness as well as developing physical prowess. In Tibet people went on walks which lasted for many days and nights that helped them to attain elevated mental states.

YOGA

Yoga itself is a system that encompasses physical, mental, emotional, and spiritual disciplines. The word yoga is derived from the Sanskrit root *yuj* which means to bind, to yoke, or union or communion. As a philosophic system, the aim of yoga is communion with the Goddess/God, a transcendent spiritual force. Yoga practices include disciplines for the body, intellect, mind, emotions, and will.

In the West, we know yoga primarily as body postures (*asanas*), breathing exercises (*pranayama*), and some meditation. These have been put together by various teachers, and have resulted in several schools of yoga. All the schools use the asanas or postures as their basis but may vary the way that they do them, the particular postures that they focus on, and the order of the asanas. They have different pranayama exercises which they stress as well as some meditation and chanting.

Some of the more common schools of yoga in the West include the following:

Integral Yoga—This was started by Swami Satchidananda and focuses primarily on Hatha yoga with some pranayama techniques, chanting, and meditation. The postures are taught in a very simple manner with various skill levels. Integral yoga is a good introduction for those beginning their yoga studies.

Kundalini Yoga—Kundalini yoga was begun by Yogi Bhajan. Many of those practicing kundalini yoga live in Sikh communities, wear white clothes and white turbans on their heads, and commit to kundalini yoga as their way of life.

Classes in kundalini yoga focus heavily on the breath which they refer to as the "breath of fire," otherwise called *kalabhati* or bellows. This is a deep breathing technique that forces the lungs to exhale and inhale large amounts of air. Many students feel that they can reach exalted states through this type of breathing.

Iyengar Yoga— B. K. S. Iyengar developed a system of yoga which stretches and reshapes the body in different ways. Iyengar's system focuses on proper alignment in the asanas. Teachers of Iyengar yoga often use straps, blankets, and other material to help a student stretch the body further. Some Iyengar yoga is taught with partners as well. The Iyengar approach is vigorous and emphasizes a balance between strength and flexibility.

Ashtanga Yoga—Ashtanga Yoga, as taught by K. Patabhi Jois, is an ancient system of yoga where each pose is linked to the next through a series of connected movements called *vinyasa*. Smooth deep breathing with focus on gaze (*dreti*) and the locks (*bandhas*) are synchronized with the movements. The postures are grouped together in progressively more advanced sequences.

TAI CHI CHU'AN

Tai Chi Chu'an or Tai Chi is a series of flowing movements done with the breath that imitate movements of nature such as those of birds, animals, clouds, and wind. The word *tai* means the "ultimate supreme," *chi* means the "ridgepole of a house," and *chu'an* means "an exercise involving the fists and boxing" as well as "to clasp." Tai Chi Chu'an translates as a type of boxing exercise that attempts to clasp or hold in harmony the yin and yang energies residing inside an individual.

Tai Chi involves a series of movements done in sequence that places the body in various poses, synchronizing the breath and quieting the mind. The sequence of movements is based on the polarity of the body—if the right foot moves forward, the left foot moves back, a forward or side movement is always followed by a backward movement or movement to the other side. Each Tai Chi routine consists of passive and active elements—stillness and movement, curved and straight, contraction and expansion, exhalation and inhalation, closed and open, left and right, backwards and forwards, settling and floating.

There is a long form of Tai Chi, which incorporates all the movements, and a shorter form which takes less time to learn. The number of movements used is not important, but the concentration and focus one has while performing them is what brings about the benefits of Tai Chi.

There are many benefits to be obtained from practicing Tai Chi. People who are older and who have cardiovascular problems are able to do Tai Chi because of its slow gentle movements. One acquires balance and coordination

from these movements; circulation and blood flow is increased while digestion and lung capacity are improved. There is more mental clarity with a
greater ability to focus and concentrate. Because of more chi flowing through
the organs, there are fewer energy blocks and less occurrences of disease.

CHI GUNG (CHI GONG OR QIGONG)

Chi Gung focuses on simple exercises and breathing to increase the supply of
chi, ease its flow, and build stamina while achieving mental control. During
these exercises, it is common to feel various sensations as the chi moves
through the body; heat, pressure, and tingling sensations are the most frequent. During practice, many may also experience trembling or pain in certain areas of the body.

While it may take a while for the healing effects of Chi Gung to manifest
themselves—after each session one feels more alert, energetic, centered, and
peaceful. In advanced practice, an adept can mentally direct the flow of chi to
various parts of the body, and even—to a certain extent—outside of the body.
Skilled Chi Gung practitioners are often called upon to help cure those who are
ill. This is because they are able to feel the specific imbalances or stagnations in
the chi of others. Practitioners may use their own chi in balancing others.

Traditional Chinese martial artists all study Chi Gung. This is because
they need to learn to direct the chi to parts of their bodies so they can decrease
the injuries caused by the blows of their opponents. They can also increase the
flow of chi to their own hands and thus be more effective when they strike.

MARTIAL ARTS

There are many forms of *martial arts*—aikido, judo, karate, kung fu, tae kwan
do—but their essence is similar. Weaponless forms of combat existed in China
in the days of Huang Ti, the "Yellow Emperor," whose army used them in battle as long ago as 2674 B.C.E. Most scholars believe that the ancient precursors
of the martial arts were developed by Bodhidharma, an Indian monk who
arrived in China about 520 A.D.

Some of the sources that led to the martial arts are ancient Indian and
Chinese weaponless fighting, Buddhism and its nonviolent philosophy, yoga
exercises and movements, I-Ching and its principles of harmonizing with
change, and Taoism with its breathing exercises.

The martial arts were originally called *kung fu* in China. (*Kung* means
"master" and *fu* means "man," so *kung fu* is a master of man.) *Karate* developed in Okinawa in the 17th century as an outgrowth of the Japanese subju-
gation of the island and the prohibition of weapons; (*kara te*) means ("empty
hand"). *Aikido* developed in Japan along with Zen Buddhism in the 19th cen-

tury. *Judo* is an outgrowth of the ancient art of *jujitsu*, which was created by Professor Jigor Kan in Japan in 1882.

The object of the martial arts is to defend oneself and to overcome another without the use of any weapons but instead through the mastery of many movements and forms along with one's own skill and resourcefulness. A student of the martial arts is taught various stances and then works with a partner in developing strength and mastering different situations. Breath is an important part of the training since deep breathing empties the mind of thought and allows the chi to flow through the body. The body is kept very soft and relaxed with deep breathing until the moment of impact, and then certain sets of muscles are contracted.

Practicing any of the martial arts strengthens not only the body but also the mind; practitioners receive insights into the psychological mechanisms that they use when there is danger or when it is necessary to handle a difficult situation. Reflexes are sharpened and actions become more defined. After practicing Aikido many years ago, I felt that I became a better automobile driver, quicker and more concise in my actions.

AEROBIC EXERCISE

Aerobic exercise makes the heart work more efficiently and increases the blood's oxygen-carrying capacity. When the heart is able to pump blood with less effort, it has more time to rest between beats. One is able to exercise for longer periods without getting tired. Aerobic exercise creates new blood vessels, which helps to prevent heart disease when some of the existing arteries are clogged with plaque. Aerobic exercise also lengthens blood clotting time, lowers blood pressure, and prevents gout by lowering uric acid levels.

There are many types of aerobic exercise. The most common is generally referred to as "aerobics," which consists of exercises done to music that involve different movements of the legs and feet, and arms and torso. Each set of exercises is repeated several times, and then the pace is increased. Usually there is a warm-up and various stretches before the aerobics begin. Every few sets of exercises one often stops to take a pulse rate. By doing this, one can tell the effect of the aerobics on the heart. There is often a cooldown at the end of the series.

Dance aerobics usually involves more complex steps and movements but the principles are the same. Other forms of aerobic exercise are walking, jogging, and running. Aerobic walking or speed walking, is walking at a fast pace to increase the circulation or heart rate. Many people set a goal of a few miles that they cover in a certain time period and may check their pulse when finished. After using walking as an aerobic activity, one often begins to jog. Joggers need to do warm-up stretches, especially for the knees, which are a sensitive area. They also need to wear the right kind of shoes, as do runners. Jogging and running can provide a tremendous release of tension, as well as a kind of euphoria or high. The flow of epinephrine (often mistaken for adrenaline) is increased, a hormone that causes a surge of energy to the brain. Swimming is another exercise that may be done aerobically; one swims so many laps in a certain time period to increase the heart rate. Aerobic exercise is especially important in the winter when the body is cooler and circulation is sluggish.

DANCE THERAPY

Through the ages, dance has provided a release of physical and emotional energies as well as opening the door to more transcendent states of consciousness. In Asia there have been the trance dances of Bali; in the Arabic countries, the Whirling Dervishes; in African and Native American tribal cultures, all-night dances performed with drums and other instruments.

Western therapeutic dance was begun by Rudolph Laban (1879–1959). Laban started with theater dance in Germany, but then fled to England during the war where he worked with freer movements to create better emotional and mental states. Dance therapy is used with many psychiatric patients to help them express their emotions and achieve a better balance between body and mind.

FELDENKRAIS AND ALEXANDER TECHNIQUE
(Included in the Somatics section in Chapter 4.)

CONCLUSION: DIAGNOSTIC TECHNIQUES

Any symptom or imbalance can be caused by a number of Paracelsus' causes of disease in combination. This can make it difficult to determine which alternative healing technique would be most appropriate for a particular condition. For example, should one focus on the flow of *chi*, or on whether certain vertebrae in the back are out?

A variety of diagnostic techniques can help a healer determine which causes should be addressed first, and thus which therapies might be most appropriate. Most of these diagnostic techniques encompass the psycho/spiritual level, the psychological level, and the physiological level. Some of the techniques are broader than others. A particular healer or practitioner will no doubt choose the diagnostic tool that has an affinity with the healing modality being used.

For myself as a healer, I tend to use two techniques. The first is Astrology because I am a Medical Astrologer and have been using this modality very successfully for many years. Studying the astrological horoscope through the planetary transits shows me what is happening *now* and which organs or systems might be involved. The horoscope also shows me what is going on psychologically and spiritually with the person that could be related to these symptoms. After I glean this information, I do some dowsing, which is an easy and quick technique to do. The dowsing confirms that these particular organ systems are involved, and will also help me to determine which physical remedies, such as herbs and nutritional supplements, are called for, as well as which homeopathic remedy. The dowsing acts as a confirming tool even when you feel you already know the remedy. I also use dowsing to check out any practitioners such as acupuncturists, bodyworkers or colonic therapists that might be helpful for my client.

Another very complete diagnostic tool is Iridology; in studying the iris, one can see psychological temperaments as well as weak systems in the physical body. Other healers start with pulse diagnosis to see which organs are weak and whether the chi needs balancing. Some bodyworkers use feet and toes to see which pressure points are sensitive and sore. Many practitioners of Traditional Chinese Medicine use facial diagnosis in addition to examining the pulses and tongue.

An example of how these techniques might be used is illustrated by how I treated a condition I recently experienced. I started getting numbness and soreness on my right leg above the knee that went to the thigh area. Later, I got occasional nerve spasms that started in the area and went through my entire leg. Knowing what was happening in my astrological chart, I increased magnesium, manganese, and B-complex vitamins, which are all essential to the nervous system. I also drank some St. John's wort tea (St. John's wort is an herb that helps to balance the nervous system), made compresses of St. John's wort oil for my leg, and took a dose of homeopathic Hypericum (a remedy made from the herb St. John's wort which works with the higher nervous system). Since I was seeing a neuromuscular therapist weekly, I told him about the condition. He found that it was related to a certain nerve whose origin was in the sacrum as well as a condition in my right hip. After he worked on it for several weeks, the nerve condition disappeared but the numbness was still there. This corresponded to what was happening in my chart again—the Uranus transits, which relate to the higher nervous system—were not as close now, but I was under two Saturn transits. Saturn can indicate inhibition and blockage. Because Saturn was sitting on my Jupiter for a few months, I examined this symbolism. Jupiter rules the liver and pancreas; Saturn the gallbladder. It would seem that there was some blockage in my liver or gallbladder though I had no symptoms in either organ. When I went to my acupuncturist, she saw that the numbness was on the gallbladder meridian. After one acupuncture treatment, the condition was almost totally alleviated.

An explanation of the major diagnostic techniques in complementary medicine follows.

This one example involved several different diagnoses—Medical Astrology, dowsing, determination of nerve plexes by the neuromuscular therapist, as well as pulse and meridian diagnosis by my acupuncturist. This could have happened in a different sequence, but obviously I was supposed to learn some new material regarding the nerve plexes as well as have some deep work done on my right hip, which had been out for a long time. The spiral of healing is always different even if the condition is similar. Since all imbalance is an opportunity for us to go deeper into our own psyches and bodies, each time we have an imbalance we learn something new.

IRIDOLOGY

Iridology is the science that analyzes the iris of the eye in order to determine physical constitution, tissue weakness, and psychological traits. The iris is the portion of the eye that carries the color. (Iris was the goddess of the rainbow in Greek mythology.) The fibers of the iris comprise a huge communication network, since the iris is connected to every organ and tissue by way of the brain and nervous system. The nerve fibers receive their impulses through connections to the optic nerve, the optic thalami, and the spinal cord. The eye, therefore, not only enables us to bring images of the outside world within, it also shows images of what is within our bodies and psyches to the outside world.

Iridology dates back to the early 1800s when a young Hungarian, Ignatz von Peczely, caught an owl in his garden. While struggling with the owl, he accidentally broke its leg. When he looked into the owl's eyes, he saw a black stripe appear. As he nursed it back to health, the black stripe was replaced by white lines. Years later, von Peczely became a doctor and observed changes in his patients' eyes after accidents, surgeries, and illnesses. He created the first chart of the iris based on these findings.

Modern iridology was pioneered by Dr. Bernard Jensen, who developed a map of the iris that represents the placement of organs and tissues. The iris is divided into seven zones; the right iris is comparable to the right side of the body; the left, to the left side. There are 90 known specific areas on each iris (see page 138) and each iris is different.

When observing the iris, the first impression is of its overall appearance—how light or dark it is, its color, whether there are any black holes or lesions on it. This gives an idea of constitutional strength.

Colored spots on the eye can be psora and/or drug deposits. *Psora* are heavy dark patches which are usually inherited. Drug spots are smaller and different in color. Chemical deposits—including those from drugs—show up as bright yellow, red, orange, and other colors. They are usually scattered about and found mostly in the digestive zone and the glandular zone.

By observing the shape of the pupil and its size, it is possible to learn where major stresses are occurring in the body. The pupil is not located in the center of the iris. It is slightly down from the geometric center. If it is small and pinched down, a condition of extreme nervous tension is indicated. When it is wide and open beyond its usual perimeter, a condition of nerve depletion and exhaustion is present. The response to light is also an indication of tension or stress.

On the map of the iris, the digestive system is the hub, the stomach being in the first area and the intestines in the second (see page 139). This is because all nutrients that sustain body tissue are obtained from the results of the

CHART TO IRIDOLOGY

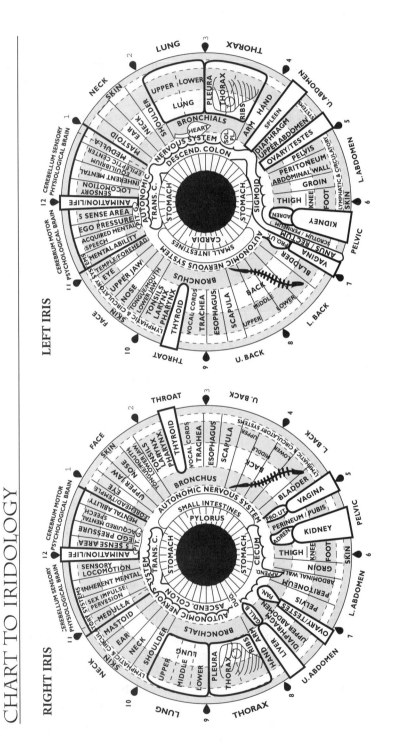

LEFT IRIS

RIGHT IRIS

Iridology Chart developed by Dr. Bernard Jensen, D.C. © 1948

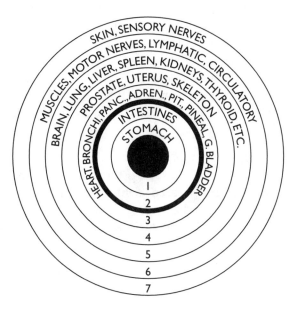

The iris is divided into 7 zones.

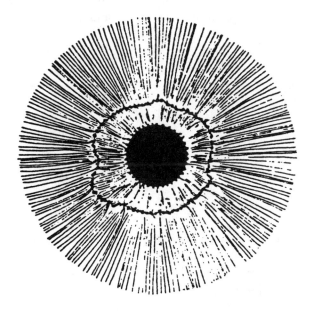

The autonomic nerve wreath is a major landmark.

digestive process. The second zone is usually darker than other parts of the iris as this is where the greatest amount of toxicity is found. Dark areas on the colon usually indicate pockets or diverticula that do not remove waste materials very well. It is easy for infections to get started here. Often a change of diet and cleansing will help to remove these pockets.

Healing can be observed through the iris when white lines come forth. Healing lines often appear in the intestinal area and lead to healing in other areas.

Method of Analysis

To make an accurate analysis, an iridologist photographs each iris. These can be compared with photographs taken later for signs of healing and change. A transparent overlay of the iris chart is placed over the photograph of each iris and correspondences made. An iridologist will also make a personal observation of the irises with a magnifying glass and a light.

MEDICAL ASTROLOGY

The astrological horoscope is one of the oldest diagnostic tools in both the Eastern and Western worlds. Hippocrates, the father of modern medicine, stated, "A physician without a knowledge of astrology cannot rightly call himself a physician." Following the Hermetic axiom, "As above, so below," Hippocrates contended that one could not know the disposition and temperament of an individual without an understanding of the greater environment in which the person was born.

Certain planetary configurations dispose us to have weaknesses in particular organs in our body which correspond to emotional states. By being aware of these areas, we can work not only with our psychological patterns but also with physical exercise, diet, herbs, and supplements to maintain our bodies in a state of vitality and health.

Understanding the cycles of the planets can also show us why we may lack certain minerals or vitamins at particular time periods and when these time periods occur. Thus, we can work preventively to maintain ourselves in a state of physiological and psychological balance.

What to Look for in the Horoscope:

1. First look at the *Sun* and its aspects (distances from other planets). The Sun shows the constitutional vitality and vigor. Its aspects to other planets indicate metabolic tendencies—whether one burns energy quickly or slowly.

2. The *Moon* is the "amperage"—how the vital forces flow through the body. Certain types of aspects from the Moon may make the individ-

ual ill from time to time though the vital force may be strong. This indicates a need for more rest and slowing down.

3. The *Ascendant* or rising sign is the conductor of energy. Fire and Air signs are the strongest conductors, Earth and Water are less strong. This can be changed if a strong Fire planet like Mars is near one of the angles of the chart. One may be more physically sensitive if a Water planet like the Moon or Neptune is near one of the angles.

4. The element balance in the horoscope should be studied. In determining the element balance, the planets and houses are considered as well as the signs. The first, fifth, and ninth houses are Fire houses; second, sixth, and tenth are Earth; third, seventh, and eleventh—Air; and fourth, eighth, and twelfth—Water. The Sun, Mars, and Jupiter are Fire planets; Saturn, Earth; Mercury and Uranus—Air; Moon, Venus, and Neptune—Water. Pluto may be considered a combination of Fire and Water. When these planets are angular or in close hard aspect to the Sun and Moon, they may balance other factors in the horoscope.

With a lack of planets in Fire signs (Aries, Leo, Sagittarius), there is less physical vitality and a tendency to lethargy and depression. These individuals need much physical exercise. A preponderance of planets in Fire indicates a person who often burns out, not conserving physical energy. These people are constantly on the go and rarely take time to reflect on life.

A lack of the Earth element (Taurus, Virgo, Capricorn) frequently leads one to ignore the physical body. Often these individuals have pale, sensitive skin, unless they spend enough time outdoors. An abundance of the Earth element usually indicates those who enjoy taking care of their physical needs by exercising, cooking, and other activities. Sometimes they tend to be too focused on their physical bodies, especially with a strong Virgo or sixth house emphasis.

Lack of the Air element (Gemini, Libra, Aquarius) may point to a weak nervous system and difficulty in communicating. Many planets in Air tend to make one mentally active. These people habitually overdo mental projects and often develop symptoms that relate to the nervous system and respiratory ailments. Working with yoga, exercise, and breathing techniques can be very helpful for them.

Individuals having few planets in Water (Cancer, Scorpio, Pisces) may find difficulty expressing emotions; they also tend to lack fluids in the body. If this is not balanced out, toxins may accumulate. Drinking more liquids and frequent juice fasts are helpful. With an excess of the Water element, emotionally caused conditions are prominent. These individuals are supersensitive and tend to absorb negative feelings from others as well. They need to learn detachment from personal feelings.

5. The next thing to consider is planetary placement in Cardinal, Fixed, and Mutable signs, and in Angular, Succedent, and Cadent houses (which correspond to Cardinal, Fixed, and Mutable signs). *Cardinal* signs (Aries, Cancer, Libra, and Capricorn) relate to body structure, the gastrointestinal system, the eyes, and the kidneys. With an emphasis in the Cardinal signs or Angular houses, these areas of the body may be affected. *Fixed* signs (Taurus, Leo, Scorpio, Aquarius) govern the throat and thyroid, the reproductive and excretory systems, and the heart and circulatory systems. Emphasis in the Fixed signs indicates intractability and stubbornness with a holding back of energy and retaining of toxins. These individuals need to let go of their emotions. *Mutable* signs (Gemini, Virgo, Sagittarius, Pisces) rule the nervous system. Mutable sign people tend to throw off toxins more readily and often have a faster recovery process. They are adaptable and flexible, though often indecisive and wishy-washy.

6. The emphasis of planets in one sign or one house should be noted. This usually indicates a sensitivity in the corresponding area of the body.

Physiological Meanings of the Astrological Signs

Aries/Libra—"balance"—This polarity represents the "I" of Aries and the "we" of Libra. If relationships with one's self and between others is balanced, then the body should be in balance as well. Aries rules the head that takes in oxygen and lets out carbon dioxide, Libra rules the kidneys that eliminate the liquid wastes from the body.

Taurus/Scorpio—"cleansing"—These signs feed the body as well as cleanse and purify by ridding it of waste material—Taurus through the throat, and Scorpio through the colon and excretory system. If one takes in too many negative emotions, there may be a need to cleanse the body and let go of desire and strong will.

Gemini/Sagittarius—"communication"—Gemini and Sagittarius govern the nervous system and the body's communication system. Gemini rules the arms, hands, shoulders, lungs, and nerves, while Sagittarius governs the hips, thighs, sciatic nerve, pancreas, and liver. Gemini transmits the messages and Sagittarius distributes them throughout the body. If we are under pressure—nervous or tense—our breathing may become too shallow, and we can develop problems in the area of the lungs; states of anxiety may also lead to problems with the sciatic nerve.

Cancer/Capricorn—"security-oriented"—Cancer and Capricorn provide us with the foundation and structure of our bodies. Capricorn rules the skeletal frame, bones, the teeth, cartilage, and skin; while Cancer rules the softer parts, such as the stomach, uterus, and breasts. When something goes awry in our professional work or our domestic or emotional life, it is often our body's structure that gives way with a broken bone or a slipped disc, or we develop a condition such as stomach ulcers or uterine infections in the sensitive Cancer areas.

Leo/Aquarius—"circulation"—Leo and Aquarius, creativity and the expression of it to humanity, govern circulation and oxygenation. Leo rules the heart, the center of the circulatory system, which in Aquarius sends out the energy to all the cells of the body. Aquarius also rules the ankles; swollen ankles often result from circulatory dysfunction. If we repress our feelings or block our emotions, we tend to have poor circulation (we speak of a "cold" person). Impaired circulation can lead to abnormal heart conditions.

Virgo/Pisces—"digestion and assimilation"—Virgo and Pisces are signs of health and healing; Virgo rules the intestines and the entire digestive system; Pisces governs the duodenum—the first part of the small intestine—which is prone to ulcers. Pisces also rules the lymphatic system that is comprised of cells that attack and neutralize invading bacteria. When we take on too many projects, especially of a mental nature (since Virgo is ruled by the planet Mercury), we have difficulty assimilating our experiences and often develop digestive problems.

Physiological Rulership of Planets

Sun—heart and circulatory system

Moon—fluids, mucous membranes, stomach

Mercury—nervous and respiratory systems

Venus—throat, thyroid gland

Mars—muscles, adrenal glands, blood

Jupiter—liver, pancreas

Saturn—skeletal system, teeth, bones, joints, skin, gallbladder

Uranus—nervous system along with Mercury

Neptune—cerebrospinal fluid, pineal gland, lymphatic system

Pluto—bowels, reproductive system

Physical Symptoms Associated with the Planets

Sun—cardiovascular diseases

Moon—inflammation of mucous membranes, imbalance of body fluids (edema, dehydration), digestive problems

Mercury—neuritis, respiratory ailments, impediments of speech

Venus—throat infections, thyroid imbalance, kidney problems

Mars—swelling and inflammation, fevers, infections, accidents, hemorrhage and blood diseases

Jupiter—liver diseases (hepatitis), pancreatic diseases (hypoglycemia, diabetes), obesity, abnormal growth, tumors

Saturn—arthritis, rheumatism, fractures, spinal ailments, dental problems, skin diseases, gallstones

Uranus—cramps, spasm, shock, paralysis, epilepsy, radiation poisoning

Neptune—obscure diseases, hallucinations, poisonings and overdoses, alcoholism and addictions, toxic conditions, schizophrenia

Pluto—destruction of tissue, hidden cell changes, diseases of the reproductive organs

Zodiacal Anatomy

Aries—head, face, eyes, nose

Taurus—neck, throat, mouth, tonsils, vocal cords

Gemini—arms, shoulders, lungs

Cancer—stomach, breasts, diaphragm, uterus

Leo—cardiac region, spleen, heart

Virgo—lower abdominal area, small intestine

Libra—small of back, kidneys, bladder

Scorpio—pelvis, reproductive organs, colon, rectum

Sagittarius—thighs, hips, buttocks, liver, pancreas

Capricorn—knees, bones, gallbladder, teeth, cartilage

Aquarius—calves, ankles, retina of eyes

Pisces—feet, lymphatic system

TRADITIONAL CHINESE DIAGNOSIS

(See material in Chapter 5 under The Four Examinations.)

MACROBIOTIC ORIENTAL DIAGNOSIS

In Macrobiotics, traditional Oriental diagnostic techniques are used that are similar to the Chinese system. The emphasis, however, is slightly different. It includes the taking of the pulse, facial diagnosis, as well as the study of the hands and feet, the nails, the tongue, the eyes, and the ears. Macrobiotic diagnosis takes into consideration these seven things:

1. Destiny—whether a person is or will become happy or not.
2. Personality—what are the ideals, view of life, nature and character.
3. Constitution—what is the constitution both physical and mental.
4. Disorders—what type of disorders the individual has developed and is suffering at present.
5. Recommendations—what changes are required to turn these disorders into health and well-being.
6. Orientation—what kind of future orientation should there be for the realization of happiness.
7. Inspiration—what encouragement should be given to develop the possibility to achieve happiness.

In determining constitution, family, social, and cultural influences are noted—as well as the date of conception and birth since Orientals look at the astrological horoscope to see the planetary influences and what effect they have upon the individual in terms of potential health problems, mental abilities, emotional makeup, and spiritual aspirations.

To evaluate the organs, several different pulses on the wrist are examined. The ability to study the pulses and the nuances in their rhythm takes many years to develop. These are the general pulse correspondences:

right hand	1. deep: lungs surface: large intestine
	2. deep: spleen and pancreas surface: stomach
	3. deep: sex/circulation (pericardium) surface: triple burner
left hand	1. deep: heart surface: small intestine
	2. deep: liver surface: gallbladder
	3. deep: kidneys surface: bladder

After the pulses are determined, a general study of the face is made. The face and the head represent the conditions of the internal organs.

The cheeks show the condition of the lungs and their functions.

The tip of the nose represents the heart, while the nostrils represent the bronchi connecting the lungs. The middle part of the nose signifies the stomach, while the upper part reveals the condition of the pancreas.

The eyes portray the kidneys as well as the condition of the ovaries of a woman and the testicles of a man. Also, the left eye represents the spleen and pancreas, while the right eye represents the liver and gallbladder.

The area between the eyebrows shows the condition of the liver, and the temples on both sides show the condition of the spleen.

The forehead as a whole represents the small intestine, and the peripheral region of the forehead, the large intestine. The upper part of the forehead shows the condition of the bladder.

The ears represent the kidneys: the left ear, the left kidney; the right ear, the right kidney.

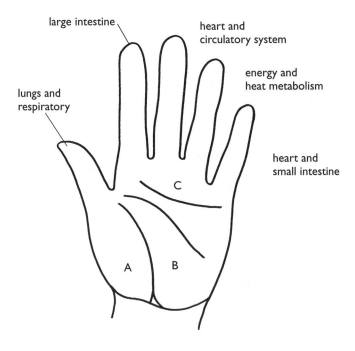

Palms and Fingers

The mouth as a whole shows the condition of the entire digestive vessel. The upper lip shows the stomach; the lower lip, the small intestines at the inner part of the lip and the large intestines at the more peripheral part of the lip. The corners of the lip show the condition of the duodenum.

The area around the mouth represents the sexual organs and their functions.

The palms and hands are also studied in assessing organ balance (see illustration on page 146).

Palms and Fingers

Line A and its related area on the palm at the base of the thumb signifies the digestive and respiratory functions, including the state of the esophagus, stomach, small intestine, large intestine, and lungs.

Line B and its area represent the nervous system, including the brain and central nervous system as well as the peripheral nerves.

Line C and the upper palm represent the circulatory and excretory systems, which include the heart, kidneys, and bladder.

The Fingers

The fingers represent the organs and functions located in the upper part of the body, namely the lungs and heart. They also are connected to the small intestine and large intestine as well as their related functions such as circulation and heat metabolism. Each finger corresponds to a certain function:

the thumb—functions of the lungs and respiratory activities

the index finger—large intestine and its functions

the middle finger—heart and circulatory functions, including reproductive vitality

the ring finger—the activity of eliminating excess energy from the regions of the heart, stomach, and intestines; energy and heat metabolism

the little finger—heart and small intestine

The Feet and Toes

Studying the feet and toes is another way to determine the condition of the organs and their functions (see illustrations on page 148).

Points A, B, and C correspond to the kidneys, heart, stomach, and the abdominal center. The inside ball of the foot (D) under the big toe corresponds to the shoulders and shoulder blades, while the outside ball (E) corresponds to the lungs and respiratory functions.

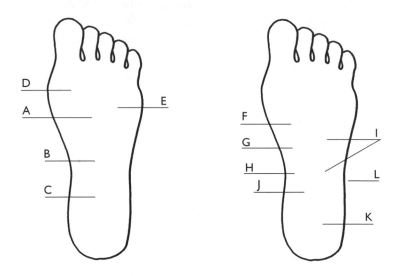

Foot—Body correlations

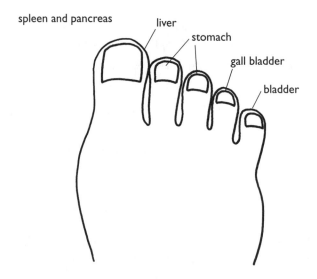

Toes—Organ correlations

The inside middle region of the foot (F) represents the nose and mouth cavity, (G) the throat and vocal cords, and (H) the bronchi and diaphragm region.

The outer middle region of the foot (I) signifies the stomach, duodenum, and upper intestinal region.

The inner lower region (J) corresponds to the intestinal region, especially the middle part of the intestines.

The heel (K) as a whole correlates to the lower intestinal region, the rectum, and the uterus.

The line running along the bottom outside of the foot (L) represents the spine and the muscles along the spine, as well as the meridian related to the bladder functions.

The toes and toenails represent the functions and the organs which are located in the middle region of the body, namely the spleen and pancreas, liver, stomach, gallbladder, and bladder.

The first toe and its nail, especially the outer area, correspond to the spleen and pancreas. At the inner area, they also correspond to the liver and its functions.

The second and third toes and their nails represent the stomach and its functions. The second toe represents the stomach organ with the third toe signifying the functions of the stomach sphincter and duodenum.

The fourth toe and its nail correspond to the gallbladder and its functions.

The fifth toe and its nail relate to the bladder and its processes.

These are just some of the ways the Oriental practitioner assesses the conditions of the body organs. The practitioner also studies the eyes, the ears, and the tongue in order to evaluate the temperament of the individual as well as the status of the organs and their functions. Then the patient can learn to balance the body and psyche in order to prepare for future goals.

MEDICAL RADIESTHESIA

Medical radiesthesia (often referred to as dowsing) is a good diagnostic tool for assessing imbalances within the various organs of the body. It is also extremely helpful in testing for food allergies, preparing herbal formulas and flower remedies, and in checking vitamin and mineral supplements.

Waves of force (commonly called *vibrations*) emanate from all objects in the physical universe and from levels of consciousness that lie beyond the range of physical sense perception. Various instruments like the dowsing rod and the pendulum have been used to detect and measure these forces. These instruments can be used by any individual who takes the time to develop this ability.

A *pendulum* or *dowsing rod* is a way of bringing higher information into conscious awareness. These tools act to amplify the neuromuscular response by providing a clear set of signals. *Witnesses* or substances symbolizing the person are often used—a photograph, a lock of hair, a blood spot, saliva, the name of the person written on a piece of paper, or an astrological chart.

When testing foods or remedies, the physical substance itself can be utilized or its name can be written on a piece of paper. The pendulum alone can be used for a yes/no or neutral valuation of the food or remedy. Further information as to how positive or negative the substance in question is can be determined by the size of the pendulum's swing.

Remedies can also be placed in the middle of a wheel with a circular scale of 360 degrees to measure their potency. The pendulum may swing close to 270 degrees for one remedy or 300 degrees for another, confirming that the second remedy is more potent.

RADIONICS

Radionics is based on the same principle as radiesthesia but uses a machine to determine the cause of disease and to project various remedies for the patient in order to restore health.

As a healing discipline, radionics developed from the research of the American physician, Dr. Albert Abrams. Abrams, who was a specialist in nervous disease, discovered that certain areas of the abdomen gave a dull note on percussion when particular diseases were present. In order to identify these disease reflexes, he devised an instrument with calibrated dials to measure intensities. In 1924, his instruments were tested in England and their diagnostic value was upheld.

Ruth Drown, an American chiropractor, developed a more sophisticated form of radionic instrumentation in the 1930s. She found that it was possible to diagnose as well as treat the disease of a patient from a distance using a sample of blood as a link. In the 1940s and 1950s, extensive research into radionics was done at Oxford, England by George and Marjorie De La Ware. In the 1970s Malcolm Rae, an American, added a new dimension through using magnetically energized geometric patterns and electronically pulsed distance treatment.

In radionics, all diseases, organs, and remedies have their own special frequency or vibration. These are expressed in numerical values known as *rates*. The radionics machine has calibrated dials upon which the frequencies or rates can be placed.

Usually, a patient sends a blood spot or hair sample to the practitioner who places that on the radionics instrument and adjusts the dials (like tuning a radio to receive a transmission). The practitioner then goes through a series of questions to get a picture of the patient's health, selecting those rates which will counteract the imbalance and then the practitioner broadcasts to the patient a homeopathic medicine, color, flower remedy, vitamin or mineral supplement. Other treatments, such as structural work or acupuncture, may be suggested as well.

One of the advantages of radionics is that it assesses the underlying causes that give rise to pathological states and prevents these from developing further.

APPLIED KINESIOLOGY

Applied kinesiology is more of a confirmation tool than a broad diagnostic technique.

Applied kinesiology uses a system of simple muscle-testing procedures to assess the energy levels in the different organs and body systems. Dr. George Goodheart, an American chiropractor, discovered that the tests used in kinesiology to determine muscle strength and tone over the range of movement of the joints could also determine the balance of energy in each of the body's systems. With further research, he established the relationship between each muscle group, the particular organs, and the acupuncture meridians.

Many chiropractors and other healers are now using applied kinesiology to discern structural imbalances, to determine dietary deficiencies and allergies, and to detect various organ dysfunctions. Once imbalances have been found by muscle testing, any treatment may be carried out and the effects monitored by repeating the muscle test and comparing the results. Muscle testing can reveal how effective the treatment has been, how often it is required, and the dosage of any remedies or supplements the body needs.

MEDICAL PALMISTRY

As was explained in the section on Oriental diagnosis, a study of the palms and the nails is an excellent tool in assessing health patterns. The coloring of the hands and nails also provides us with information on the basic vitality and circulation. The condition of particular organs can be determined by individual fingers and certain points on the palm.

BIBLIOGRAPHY

GENERAL

Airola, Paavo, N.D. *How to Get Well*. Phoenix, AZ: Health Plus, Publications, 1974.

Asimov, Isaac. *The Human Body—Its Structure and Operation*. New York: New American Library, 1963.

Ballantine, Rudolph, M.D. *Diet and Nutrition—A Holistic Approach*. Honesdale, PA: Himalayan International Institute, 1978.

A Barefoot Doctor's Manual. Seattle, WA: Madrona Publishers, Inc., 1977.

Bliss, Shepherd, ed. *The New Holistic Health Handbook: Living Well in a New Age*. Berkeley, CA: Berkeley Holistic Center, Stephen Greene Press, Inc., 1985.

Bricklin, Mark, ed. *The Practical Encyclopedia of Natural Healing*. Emmaus, PA: Rodale Press, Inc., 1983.

Carroll, David. *The Complete Book of Natural Medicines*. New York: Summit Books, 1980.

Clark, Linda. *Get Well Naturally*. New York: ARC International, Ltd., 1965.

Cousins, Norman. *Anatomy of an Illness as Perceived by the Patient*. New York: W. W. Norton & Co., Inc., 1979.

Dextreit, Raymond. *Our Earth, Our Cure*. Ed. and tr. from French by Michael Abehsera. Secaucus, NJ: Citadel Press, 1986.

Haas, Elson. *Staying Healthy with the Seasons*. Berkeley, CA: Celestial Arts Pub. Co., 1981.

Hall, Manly Palmer. *Paracelsus: His Mystical and Medical Philosophy*. Los Angeles, CA: Philosophical Research Society, 1964.

Hay, Louise. *Heal Your Body—Metaphysical Causations for Physical Illness*. Los Angeles, CA: Louise Hay, 1976.

Hay, Louise. *You Can Heal Your Life*. Santa Monica, CA: Hay House, Inc., 1988.

Heritage, Ford. *Composition and Facts about Foods*. Mokelumne Hill, CA: Health Research, 1971.

Hill, Ann, ed. *A Visual Encyclopedia of Unconventional Medicine*. New York: Crown Publishers, Inc., 1978.

Hunter, Beatrice Trum. *Consumer Beware!* Touchstone Books. New York: Simon and Schuster, Inc., 1971.

Jackson, Mildred, N.D., and Terri Teague. *The Handbook of Alternatives to Chemical Medicine*. Oakland, CA: Terri Teague and Mildred Jackson, 1974.

Jensen, Bernard. *World Keys to Health and Long Life*. Provo, UT: Bi World Industries, Inc., 1975.

Kirschmann, John D. *Nutrition Almanac.* New York: McGraw-Hill Pub. Co., 1979.

Kulvinskas, Viktoras. *Survival into the 21st Century.* Woodstock Valley, CT: Omangod Press, 1975.

Myss, Caroline Ph.D. *Anatomy of The Spirit.* Harmony Books. New York: Crown Publishers, 1996.

Reilly, Harold J., M.D. *The Edgar Cayce Handbook for Health through Drugless Therapy.* New York: Macmillan Publishing Co., Inc., 1975.

Rohe, Fred. *The Complete Book of Natural Foods.* Boulder, CO: Shambhala Publications, 1983.

Samuels, Mike, M.D., and Hall Bennett. *The Well Body Book.* New York: Random House, Inc., 1978.

Schneider, Meir. *Self-Healing: My Life and Vision.* New York & London: Routledge & Kegal Paul, Ltd., 1987.

Selye, Hans. *The Stress of Life.* New York: McGraw-Hill Pub. Co., 1956.

Siegel, Bernie, M.D. *Love, Medicine, and Miracles.* New York: Harper & Row Publications, Inc., 1990.

_____. *Peace, Love, and Healing.* New York: Harper & Row Publications, Inc., 1990.

Steadman, Alice. *Who's The Matter with Me?* Marina del Rey, CA: De Vorss & Co., 1966.

Vogel, Virgil. *American Indian Medicine.* Norman, OK: Univ. of Oklahoma Press, 1970.

Weil, Andrew. *From Chocolate to Morphine.* New York: Houghton Mifflin Co., 1993.

_____. *Health and Healing.* New York: Houghton Mifflin Co., 1983.

_____. *Natural Health, Natural Medicine.* New York: Houghton Mifflin Co., 1990.

Williams, Roger J. *Biochemical Individuality: The Basis for the Genetotrophic Concept.* Austin, TX: Univ. of Texas Press, 1956.

CHAPTER 1: VIBRATIONAL HEALING

Becker, Robert O., M.D., and Sheldon, Gary. *The Body Elecronic—Electromagnetism and the Foundation of Life.* New York: William Morrow, 1985.

Brennan, Barbara Ann. *Hands of Light: A Guide to Healing Through the Human Energy Field.* New York: Bantam, 1987.

Berendt, Joachim-Ernst. *The World is Sound—Nada Brahma.* Rochester, VT: Inner Traditions International, 1991.

Chopra, Deepak, M.D. *Quantum Healing: Exploring the Frontiers of Mind-Body Medicine.* New York: Bantam Books, Inc., 1989.

Clark, Linda. *The Ancient Art of Color Therapy.* New York: Simon & Schuster, Inc., 1975.

Color Healing: An Exhaustive Survey Compiled by Health Research from the 21 Works of the Leading Practitioners of Chromotherapy. Mokelumne Hill, CA: Health Research, 1956.

David, William. *The Harmonics of Sound, Color, & Vibration.* Marina del Rey, CA: De Vorss & Co., 1980.

Dinshah, Darius. *The Spectro-Chrome System.* Malaga, NJ: Dinshah Health Society, 1979.

Flower Essence Repertory. Nevada City, CA: Flower Essence Society, 1986.

Gerber, Richard, M.D. *Vibrational Medicine: New Choices for Healing Ourselves.* Santa Fe, NM: Bear & Co., 1988.

Gardner, Joy. *Color and Crystals.* Freedom, CA: The Crossing Press, 1988.

_____. *The Healing Voice.* Freedom, CA: The Crossing Press, 1993.

Gimbel, Theo. *Healing Through Colour.* Saffron Walden, Essex, Great Britain: C. W. Daniel Co., Ltd., 1980.

Goldman, Jonathan. *Healing Sounds—The Power of Harmonics.* Shaftesbury, Great Britain: Element Books, 1996.

Heline, Corinne. *Healing and Regeneration through Color.* Santa Barbara, CA: J. F. Rowny Press, 1968.

_____. *Healing and Regeneration through Music.* Santa Barbara, CA: J. F. Rowny Press, 1968.

Isaacs, Thelma. *Gemstones, Crystals, & Healing.* Black Mountain, NC: Lorien House, 1982.

Keyes, Laurel. *Toning: The Creative Power of the Voice.* Marina del Rey, CA: De Vorss & Co., 1964.

Keville, Kathy and Mindy Green. *Aromatherapy—A Complete Guide to the Healing Art.* Freedom, CA: The Crossing Press, 1995.

Lingerman, Hal. *The Healing Energies of Music.* Wheaton, IL: Theosophical Publishing House, 1983.

Lorusso, Julia and Joel Glick. *Healing Stoned: The Therapeutic Use of Gems & Minerals.* Albuquerque, NM: Adobe Press, 1976.

Payne, Buryl. *The Body Magnetic.* Boulder, CO: Buryl Payne, 1988.

Price, Shirley. *Practical Aromatherapy.* Wellingborough, Northamptonshire, England: Thorsons Publishers, Inc., 1983.

Raphaell, Katrina. *Crystal Enlightenment.* Vol. I. New York: Aurora Press, 1985.

_____. *Crystal Healing.* Vol. II. New York: Aurora Press, 1987.

_____. *The Crystalline Transmission.* Vol. III. Santa Fe, NM: Aurora Press, 1990.

Tame, David, *The Secret Power of Music: The Transformation of Self & Society through Musical Energy.* New York: Destiny Books, 1984.

Tisserand, Robert. *The Art of Aromatherapy.* New York: Destiny Books, 1977.

Tomatis, Alfred. *The Conscious Ear,* Berrytown, New York: Station Hill Press, 1991.

Uyldert, Mellie. *The Magic of Precious Stones.* Wellingborough, Northamptonshire, England: Thorsons Publishers, Inc., 1981.

Valnet, Jean, M.D. *The Practice of Aromatherapy: Holistic Health & Essential Oils of Flowers & Herbs.* New York: Destiny Books, 1980.

Wright, Machaelle Small. *Flower Essences.* Jeffersonton, VA: Perelandra, Ltd., 1988.

CHAPTER 2: VIBRATIONAL BODYWORK

Kaye, Anna. *Reflexology for Good Health.* No. Hollywood, CA: Hal Leighton Printing Co., 1978.

Kreiger, Dolores. *Accepting Your Power to Heal: Personal Practice of Therapeutic Touch.* Santa Fe, NM: Bear & Company, 1993.

Teegarden, Iona. *The Acupressure Way of Health—Jin Shin Do.* Tokyo: Japan Publications, Inc. 1989.

CHAPTER 3: HOMEOPATHY

Chapman, J. B., M.D. *Dr. Schuessler's Biochemistry.* London: New Era Laboratories, 1961.

Cummings, Stephen and Dana Ullman. *Everybody's Guide to Homeopathic Medicines.* Los Angeles, CA: Jeremy P. Tarcher, Inc., 1984.

Kent, J. T. *Lectures on Homeopathic Materia Medica.* New Delhi: B. Jain Publishers, 1986.

_____. *Repertory of the Homeopathic Materia Medica.* New Delhi: B. Jain Publishers, 1986.

Panos, Maesimund B., M.D., and Jane Heimlich. *Homeopathic Medicine at Home.* Los Angeles, CA: Jeremy P. Tarcher, Inc., 1980.

Smith, Trevor. *The Homeopathic Treatment of Emotional Illness.* New York: Prentice-Hall, Inc., 1987.

Ullman, Dana. *Homeopathy: Medicine for the 21st Century.* Berkeley, CA: North Atlantic Books, 1988.

Vithoulkas, George. *Homeopathy: Medicine for the New Man.* New York: Prentice-Hall, Inc., 1987.

_____. *The Science of Homeopathy.* Athens: George Vithoulkas, Athenian School of Homeopathic Medicine, 1978.

CHAPTER 4: MENTAL AND SPIRITUAL THERAPIES

Achterberg, Jeanne. *Imagery in Healing: Shamanism and Modern Medicine.* Boulder, CO: Shambhala Publications, 1985.

Benson, William. *The Relaxation Response,* New York: Morrow Publications, 1975

Brown, Barbara. *Stress and the Art of Biofeedback.* New York: Bantam Books, Inc., 1978.

Hanna, Thomas. *The Body of Life.* New York: Alfred A. Knopf, 1987.

_____. *The End of Tyranny.* San Francisco: Free Person Press, 1976.

_____. *Bodies in Revolt—A Primer in Somatic Therapy.* San Francisco: Free Person Press, 1970.

Mindell, Arnold. *Working with the Dreaming Body.* New York: Routledge and Kegan, 1986.

Murphy, Michael. *The Future of the Body.* Los Angeles: Jeremy Tarcher, 1992.

Finkelstein, Adrian, M.D. *Your Past Lives and the Healing Process.* Palatine, IL: Adrian Finkelstein, 1985.

Mason, L. John. *Guide to Stress Reduction.* Culver City, CA: Peace Press, 1980.

Moody, Raymond, M.D. *Life After Life.* New York: Bantam Books, Inc., 1975.

Pelletier, Kenneth R. *Mind as Healer, Mind as Slayer.* New York: Dell Publishing Co., 1977.

Simonton, O. Carl, Stephanie Simonton, and James Creighton. *Getting Well Again.* New York: Bantam Books, Inc., 1981.

CHAPTER 5: TRADITIONAL CHINESE MEDICINE

Bensky, Dan et al. *Chinese Herbal Medicine: Materia Medica.* Seattle, WA: Eastland Press, 1986.

Connelly, Diane M. *Traditional Acupuncture: The Law of the Five Elements.* Columbia, MD: Center for Traditional Acupuncture, 1975, 1994.

Garvey, John W., Jr. *The Five Phases of Food: How to Begin.* Newtonville, MA: Well Being Books, 1985, pamphlet.

Hsu, Dr. Hong-Yen. *How to Treat Yourself with Chinese Herbs.* Long Beach, CA: Oriental Healing Arts Institute, 1980.

Kaptchuk, Ted J. *The Web That Has No Weaver: Understanding Chinese Medicine.* New York: Congdon & Weed, 1983.

Mann, Felix. *Acupuncture—The Ancient Chinese Art of Healing and How it Works Scientifically.* New York: Random House, 1962.

Veith, Ilza, tr. *The Yellow Emperor's Classic of Internal Medicine.* Berkeley, CA: University of California Press, 1970.

CHAPTER 6: AYURVEDIC MEDICINE

Frawley, David and Vasant Lad. *The Yoga of Herbs.* Santa Fe, NM: Lotus Press, 1986.

Heyn, Birgit. *Ayurvedic Medicine.* Wellingborough, Northants, England: Thorsons Publishing Group, 1983.

Lad, Vasant. *Ayurveda: The Science of Self-Healing.* Santa Fe, NM: Lotus Press, 1984.

Svoboda, Robert. *Prakruti: Your Ayurvedic Constitution.* Albuquerque, NM: Geocom, Ltd., 1988.

CHAPTER 7: CLEANSING AND ELIMINATION

Walker, Norman W. *Colon Health: The Key to a Vibrant Life.* Prescott, AZ: Norwalk Press, 1979.

CHAPTER 8: METABOLISM AND DIET

Aihara, Herman. *Acid and Alkaline.* Oroville, CA: George Ohsawa Macrobiotic Foundation, 1980.

Cousens, Gabriel, M.D. *Spiritual Nutrition and the Rainbow Diet.* Boulder, CO: Cassandra Press, 1986.

Kelley, W. D., D.D.S. *Metabolic Typing.* Winthrop, WA: International Health Institute, 1982, pamphlet.

CHAPTER 9: DIETARY REGIMENS

Kushi, Michio. *The Book of Macrobiotics: The Universal Way of Health and Happiness.* Tokyo: Japan Publications, Inc., 1977.

Kelley, William Donald D.D.S. *One Answer to Cancer.* The Kelley Foundation, 1974.

Lappe, Frances Moore. *Diet for a Small Planet.* New York: Ballantine Books, Inc., 1975.

Wigmore, Ann. *Why Suffer?* Boston, MA: Hippocrates Institute, 1964.

CHAPTER 10: HERBOLOGY

Gladstar, Rosemary. *Herbal Healing for Women.* New York: Simon and Schuster, 1993.

_____. *The Sage Healing Ways Series.* R. Gladstar, Box 420, E. Barre, VT 06649.

Green, James. *Herbs & Health Care for Males.* Forestville, CA: Simplers Botanicals, 1987.

Grieve, M. *A Modern Herbal.* Vols. I & II. Mineola, NY: Dover Publications, Inc., 1971.

Hoffman, David. *The Holistic Herbal.* Longmead, Shaftesbury, Dorset, England: Element Books, 1989.

Hutchens, Alma R. *Indian Herbology of North America.* Windsor, Ontario, Canada: Merco, 1969.

Kloss, Jethro. *Back to Eden.* Greenwich, CT: Benedict Lust Publications, 1971.

Lucas, Richard M. *Secrets of the Chinese Herbalists.* New York: Cornerstone Library, Inc., 1979.

Lust, John. *The Herb Book.* Greenwich, CT: Benedict Lust Publications, 1974.

Moore, Michael. *Medicinal Plants of the Mountain West.* Santa Fe: NM: Museum of New Mexico Press, 1980.

Parvati, Jeannine. *Hygeia—A Woman's Herbal.* Monroe, UT: Freestone Pub. Co., 1978.

Rose, Jeanne. *Herbs and Things.* New York: Grosset and Dunlap, 1972.

Santillo, Humbart. *Natural Healing with Herbs.* Prescott Valley, AZ: Hohm Press, 1984.

Tierra, Leslie. *The Herbs of Life.* Freedom, CA: The Crossing Press, 1992.

Tierra, Michael. *Planetary Herbology.* Santa Fe, NM: Lotus Press, 1988.

_____. *The Way of Herbs.* Berkeley, CA: Unity Press, 1980.

Weiner, Michael A. *Earth Medicine, Earth Food.* New York: Collier-Macmillan, 1980.

Wood, Matthew. *Seven Herbs: Plants as Teachers.* Berkeley, CA: North Atlantic Books, 1987.

CHAPTER 11: BODYWORK THERAPIES

Feltman, John, ed. *Hands-on Healing: Massage Remedies for Hundreds of Health Problems.* Emmaus, PA: Rodale Press, Inc., 1989.

Masunaga, Shizuto and Waturu Ohashi. *Zen/Shiatsu: How to Harmonize Yin and Yang for Better Health.* Tokyo: Japan Publications, Inc., 1977.

CHAPTER 12: EXERCISE

Feldenkrais, Moshe. *Awareness through Movement: Health Exercises for Personal Growth.* New York: Harper & Row Publications, Inc., 1972.

Iyengar, B. K. S. *Light on Yoga.* New York: Schocken Books, 1977.

Man-ch'ing, Cheng and Robert Smith. *T'ai-Chi.* Tokyo: John Weatherhill Inc., 1966.

Pritikin, Nathan. *The Pritikin Program for Diet & Exercise.* New York: Bantam Books, Inc., 1979.

Russell, W. Scott. *Karate: The Energy Connection.* New York: Delacorte Press, 1976.

Sivananda, Swami Radha. *Hatha Yoga: The Hidden Language.* Boulder, CO: Shambhala Publications, 1989.

Taylor, Louise and Betty Bryant. *Acupressure, Yoga, and You.* Tokyo: Japan Publications, Inc., 1984.

Vishnudevananda, Swami. *The Complete Illustrated Book of Yoga.* New York: Bell Publishing Co., 1960.

CONCLUSION: DIAGNOSTIC TECHNIQUES

Blackburn, Gabriele. *The Science and Art of the Pendulum: A Complete Course in Radiesthesia.* Ojai, CA: Idylwild Books, 1983.

Fairchild, Dennis. *The Handbook of Humanistic Palmistry.* Ferndale, MI: Thumbs Up, 1980.

Jensen, Bernard. *Iridology Simplified.* Bernard Jensen, Iridologists International, Route 1, Escondido, CA, 1980.

Kushi, Michio. *How to See Your Health: The Book of Oriental Diagnosis.* Tokyo: Japan Publications, Inc., 1980.

Neilsen, Greg and Joseph Polansky. *Pendulum Power.* New York: Warner Destiny Books, 1977.

Starck, Marcia. *Astrology, Key to Holistic Health.* Birmingham, MI: Seek-it Publications, 1982.

_____. *Healing with Astrology.* Freedom, CA: The Crossing Press, 1997.

Tansley, David, D.C. *Radionics & the Subtle Anatomy of Man.* Devon, England: Health Science Press, 1972.

Westlake, Aubrey, M.D. *The Pattern of Health.* Boulder, CO: Shambhala Publications, 1973.

INDEX

RELATED BOOKS FROM THE CROSSING PRESS

Healing with Astrology
By Marcia Starck
Bring balance and energy to your life using the correspondences between your horoscope and a wide range of natural healing systems—including herbs, gemstones, flower remedies, and aromatherapy.
$14.95 • Paper • 0-89594-862-1

Healing with Color Zone Therapy
By Joseph Corvo and Lilian Verner-Bonds
Corvo and Verner-Bonds introduce a form of therapy that treats the whole person: the physical, the emotional, and the spiritual. The safe, step-by-step techniques of Color Zone Therapy are followed by an A-Z list of charts for more than one hundred common ailments,
$14.95 • Paper • 0-89594-925-3

Healing with Chinese Herbs
By Lesley Tierra
Tierra lists the properties and therapeutic uses of over one hundred herbs. Includes a glossary of Chinese terms, an index to the Latin and Mandarin names of each herb, and guidelines to dosages.
$14.95 • Paper • 0-89594-829-X

Healing with Flower and Gemstone Essences
By Diane Stein
Instructions for choosing and using flowers and gems are combined with descriptions of their effect on emotional balance. Includes instructions for making flower essences and for matching essences to hara line chakras for maximum benefit.
$14.95 • Paper • 0-89594-856-7

Healing with Gemstones and Crystals
By Diane Stein
More than 200 gemstones and their healing properties are listed. Details on how to choose and use the Earth's precious gems are supplemented by explanations of the significance of this type of healing.
$14.95 • Paper • 0-89594-831-1

Essential Reiki: A Complete Guide to an Ancient Healing Art
By Diane Stein
This bestseller includes the history of Reiki, hand positions, giving treatments, and the initiations. While no book can replace directly received attunements, *Essential Reiki* provides everything else that the practitioner and teacher of this system needs, including all three degrees of Reiki, most of it in print for the first time.
$18.95 • Paper • 0-89594-736-6

The Natural Remedy Book for Women
By Diane Stein
This bestselling, self-help guide to holistic health care includes information on ten different natural healing methods. Remedies from all ten methods are given for fifty common health problems.
$16.95 • Paper • 0-89594-525-8

All Women Are Healers: A Comprehensive Guide to Natural Healing
By Diane Stein
Stein's bestselling book on natural healing for women teaches women to take control of their bodies and lives and offers a wealth of information on various healing methods including Reiki, Reflexology, Polarity Balancing, and Homeopathy.
$14.95 • Paper • 0-89594-409-X

The Male Herbal: Health Care for Men & Boys
By James Green
This preventive health care guide offers remedies for specific male problems, information on choosing the right herb, and preparation of herbal medicines.
"A wealth of information—recommended for alternative health care collections."
—*Library Journal*

$14.95 • Paper • 0-89594-458-8

Aromatherapy: A Complete Guide to the Healing Art
By Kathi Keville and Mindy Green
This complete guide presents everything you need to know to enhance your health, beauty, and emotional well-being through the practice of aromatherapy. Kathi Keville and Mindy Green offer a fresh perspective on the most fragrant of the healing arts.
$16.95 • Paper • 0-89594-692-0

The Herbs of Life: Health & Healing Using Western & Chinese Techniques
By Lesley Tierra
"This book is an herbalist's delight! It combines Western, Chinese, and Ayurvedic tradition with emphasis on energy patterns of illness and corresponding energies of herbs and food."
—The American Herb Association
$16.95 • Paper • 0-89594-498-7

To receive a current catalog from The Crossing Press,
please call toll-free, 800-777-1048.
Visit our Website on the Internet at: www.crossingpress.com